You Are In Charge!
Life, Health And Cancer

FRED BOMONTI D.C.

TO

My Parents Fred and Jean Bomonti

My spiritual teacher Rev. M. McBride Panton

My professional mentor Lee E. Arnold, D.C.

FRED BOMONTI

ENDORSEMENTS

It has been my privilege to have known Dr. Fred Bomonti for the past 50 years. He has always been a thinker and a person who could articulate his thoughts in ways that made sense to others. Now, Dr. Bomonti has authored a text that I believe should be in the library of all people, not just those who have been diagnosed with some type of cancer. His wisdom is clearly transferred to the pages of this book in a way that anyone can read and understand, and the message he brings is one of life sustaining hope for those who have received a diagnosis of some kind of significant illness. The message is not limited to concerns for the physical well-being of the reader, but extends to the mental and spiritual aspects as well because as Dr. Bomonti clearly understands, human beings cannot be segmented. We are total beings and any effort to live a healthy life, regardless of its length must consider the totality of health. I know you will enjoy and benefit by your reading of this fine book!

James Winterstein, DC, LLD (hc)

President Emeritus

National University of Health Sciences

Lombard, Illinois

Dr. Bomonti has given us a well-needed book designed to help those who have been diagnosed with cancer. Rather than advising the person to simply do what the physician or surgeon tells them to do, Dr. Bomonti offers a comprehensive method for dealing with the cancer. He doesn't solve the cancer question by offering random tidbits of advice. Rather, he offers action steps with a means of chronicling those actions to gauge adherence and progress with any given action. His is not a "one-size-fits-all" formula, but looks at monitoring progress and making appropriate corrections if a given regimen doesn't seem to be working. Unlike the medical profession, Dr. Bomonti doesn't just look at the cancer, but also analyzes the environment with which that cancer is making its home.

Whether it be a nutritional issue, a spiritual issue, stress and emotional problems, family or work issues, or the outside environment in which we live, Dr. Bomonti demands that you analyze your own personal world, and change those factors that are destructive to your well-being or recovery from cancer.

I write this as a surgical oncologist (cancer surgeon), who has worked with Dr. Bomonti on a number of perplexing cancer cases. Dr. Bomonti kindly brings up those issues which conventional medicine rarely addresses, yet are still relevant in gaining control over a cancer. To treat with alternative therapy alone is often unsuccessful. Conversely, limiting oneself to conventional medicine can be equally unsuccessful. Working together, conventional doctors and holistic physicians, a much happier balance can be achieved. Whether one is having a major surgery, radiation, or toxic chemotherapy, one usually does better if they have taken charge of the "other" aspects of their life that Dr. Bomonti so skillfully and poignantly describes in this book. Even if you don't accept everything that Dr. Bomonti has to say, this book will still be of value to you in working your own way, or that of a loved one or friend, through the quagmire of cancer treatment. I wish that many of my patients would read and act on the advice that Dr. Bomonti offers in this book.

Kenneth A. Feucht, M.D., Ph.D., FACS

PREFACE

This book is about you being in charge of your health and your future; not a doctor, the media, or your fears. Just by taking charge of, being responsible for, and taking action toward your own recovery, you have already improved your body's ability to return to good health. I refer to cancer throughout this book as a "point of reference," but the underlying causes for most cancer syndromes are the same as they are for most chronic lifestyle conditions that afflict so many in Western civilization today. Just plug in your health concern where you see a reference to cancer.

You need to know from the outset that I have been a Doctor of Chiropractic for over 45 years, and that during this time I have experienced the effects of political medicine's more than twenty-five year attempt to "contain and eliminate" the chiropractic profession with lies, misinformation, and half-truths. After many years of participating in my profession's "battles" against political medicine, I have grown to appreciate that most medical physicians are caring and dedicated professionals who often provide amazing services to their patients. However, it is apparent that many of these good people have been misinformed and misled by the political arm of their profession in regard to alternative care and alternative care providers.

Of course, because of my training (and these experiences), I have a bias in favor of the alternative perspective of health and healthcare, and I am skeptical of most medical practices, in general. I mention this in the spirit of full disclosure to help you understand some of the underlying viewpoints that have shaped my conclusions today. I do not believe that this bias changes my primary message to you, the reader, as the message is not about procedures and therapies as much as it is about you taking charge of your health and your life.

I hope you will find the information in this book useful and helpful on your journey to better health. – Fred Bomonti, DC, October 2014

LIFE NEVER RUNS OUT OF CURVEBALLS. – ANN HESSION

FRED BOMONTI

CONTENTS

FRED BOMONTI

ACKNOWLEDGMENTS

I am grateful for the encouragement of a number of people who have made this little book possible. Dr. Kenneth Feucht, M.D., Ph.D., who was my surgeon and became my friend, was the primary impetus to write something for other people going through the diagnosis of "cancer." This book would not have happened without his push, his skills and his support. In addition to Dr. Feucht's initial push, the information gained from Dr. Neil McKinney and Dr. Mark Gignac on what to do to help solve this issue was obviously "lifesaving." My good friends Dr. Jack Kornberg, Dr. Dennis Dilday, Dr. George Kurkuin, David Matteson and Charlene Hutchins each gave invaluable editorial help in reading through and offering suggestions, insights, and corrections. Dr. Russell Kolbo, my friend and physician has been there from the beginning and I don't believe I would be here sharing with you without his guidance, assistance, friendship and professional care. Thanks Russ. Ann Hession, my coach, has been invaluable in helping me to put into words my rambling thoughts and keeping me on the path to get this book written, which has been no easy task. Thanks also to Raine Dinale and Marianne Costello who have provided technical skills that have helped to get the work edited and published and to Rand Refrigeri for his talent in creating our illustrations and cover.

Finally, thank you to my wife, Jan, in encouraging me and being there to keep me focused and to say the things I needed to hear to make this little book more readable and understandable. I love you.

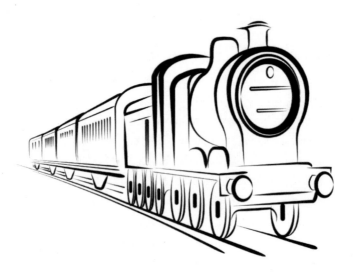

1 TRAINS

We all have heard the cliché about seeing "the light at the end of the tunnel," and I am sure most of us have heard that seemingly cynical comeback, "the light at the end of the tunnel is just another train." To me, this is not cynical but the way life works; one train after another, until we get out of the tunnel onto the other side of the mountain we call life. Changes and challenges (or what I call "trains") are inevitable, but most of us don't like change, despite knowing that change is necessary for us to grow.

My theory that we don't like change is supported by an observation that most of the advances we've made in our lifetimes were usually preceded by some kind of challenge––a crash, illness, pain, perceived failure, or defeat––forcing us to change. I visualize this process of change as if we are traveling through life in our own private locomotive, on our own set of tracks, continually getting bumped off the tracks by oncoming trains (challenges and situations). The good news in this scenario is that between trains––when the track ahead is lit from the light of another approaching train––we can get a glimpse of what may be coming next. We can plan, take action, and move forward a little...until we're knocked off again. We then pull ourselves back onto the tracks and move forward, once again into the dim light of the next train.

Getting back "on the track" is what usually takes the most time, as we are often disoriented by the last blow life has dealt us. Sometimes it seems as if we have to wander in the darkness for a while as a longer freight train passes, or until we can get a handle on our last life-challenging event. The disorientation and floundering about in the darkness we go through is why it is so important that we have goals, dreams, and a purpose for our lives.

Having a purpose in life, a direction you want to go in, things you want to accomplish, and clearly-defined goals, work together to help you refocus while in the darkness, and they can keep you from going off on a "siding" or unwanted track. Additionally, you may find that it's easier to "get back on track" to accomplishing your goals, achieving your dreams, and fulfilling your purpose, when you have a coach to help you focus. A coach can help you get your train back on the tracks and moving forward again with your life. If you are reading this book, you (or someone you know) have probably been "knocked off your tracks" and you may be wandering around in "the dark."

I write this book with the hope of helping you to regain your direction, and your life. – F.W.Bomonti, D.C.

2 INTRODUCTION

All of the animals, excepting man, know that the principal
business of life is to enjoy it. – Samuel Butler

If you are reading this book you (or someone you know) have probably been told
that you have some type of life-altering condition, like cancer or another
distressing dis-ease. Literally or figuratively speaking, your jaw dropped, your
mind has gone blank, you have raced over every possible alternative to what you
think you may have heard, and now you are probably just a little dazed. If it's a
non-cancer syndrome, you might just be relieved to now have a name for the
symptoms you've been experiencing. Either way, it is unsettling to know that this
diagnosis could very well be the cause of your death, that you are not invincible or
immortal, and that your demise no longer seems that far away or a distant
improbability. Understand that this dazed, unsettled feeling can last a while. Our
mortality is not something most of us have seriously considered until now. This
troublesome diagnosis can make our passing seem more immediate, and a real
possibility.

Some of you reading this may not have had a name or diagnosis for your
syndrome for a long time. You may have been like Moses, wandering through the
desert for a number of years, searching for an answer to the question, *what is*
wrong with me? Now that you have your diagnosis, you are faced with the
question, *what am I going to do* and *how do I handle this unwanted physical*
situation?

In his book, *The War of Art*, author Steven Pressfield paraphrased Tom Laughlin, a psychologist who primarily treats cancer patients, when he wrote:

> *"The moment a person learns he's got terminal cancer, a profound shift takes place in his psyche. At one stroke in the doctor's office, he becomes aware of what really matters to him. Things that sixty seconds earlier had seemed all-important, suddenly appear meaningless, while people and concerns that he had until then dismissed, at once take on supreme importance."*

I was diagnosed with Stage III malignant melanoma in May of 2011. Prior to this time, I knew little about melanoma, and as many do, I had included it in the same category as other skin cancers; like squamous cell and basal cell carcinoma. While all three are skin cancers, malignant melanoma is more aggressive and less treatable than the other two. Contrary to popular belief, melanoma is not necessarily related to sun or UV (ultraviolet light) exposure. Many cases are discovered in areas of the body where "the sun doesn't shine" like the bottom of the feet, between toes, and even in the rectum. For melanoma, no significant medical treatments have been shown to be especially effective, other than when the disease is discovered and treated in the earliest stages.

As this is being written, YERVOY® (generic ipilimumab, the latest medical drug treatment), has been reported to have, optimistically, 7 to 10 percent response rate for melanoma. (1) What this means is that after a year of taking medication, suffering flu-like symptoms, and enduring a financial cost of around $160,000.00, approximately 7–10 percent of patients who undergo treatment will only live three to five months beyond the average survival rate of six months to five years, and this is considered a "good" outcome. However, you may have been given a more (or less) encouraging option for your syndrome. (**Note:** With early detection, Stage I melanoma survival rates are much higher and a normal life span can be achieved.)

In my case, I was fortunate to be referred to a surgeon who is an M.D. with a Ph.D. in Anatomy. I consider myself lucky because this doctor's area of study was melanoma, and he has stayed current on the latest interventions for melanoma and how effective (or ineffective) these therapies might be. He has been honest and forthright with me, telling me since my first visit that the prognosis for people with melanoma can be one to five years, or six months, or even ten years. The diagnosis you have been given may have a different prognosis. However, all of the conditions we are considering have premature death as an option; some are just sooner than others.

For most of us who have melanoma, cancer, or an immune syndrome, nobody knows anything for sure. My doctor encouraged me to follow my alternative, vitalistic experience in caring for my body and immune system because as he informed me, there is nothing in the medical armamentarium more effective. As I write this today, I am ahead of the statistics in melanoma life expectancy.

I tell you the above so that you know what I have been through and that I am going through similar processes and experiences to what you are probably going through now. I am not sharing with you from the position of a detached academic. Instead, *I know the reality* and the feeling of finality a person can have when experiencing these conditions.

With few exceptions, and barring an intervening other cause of death, a large number of people who have been diagnosed with cancer will eventually die from the effects of that cancer, the conventional treatment for the cancer, secondary conditions caused by the treatment, or cancers caused by the treatment. With melanoma, few individuals live past 20 or more years with no symptoms and cancer free before it reappears again with fatal consequences. I am told that the good news in regard to melanoma is that it usually has a rapid decline. (Oh, boy!) However, I was not and I am not interested in *other people's outcomes*. I am interested in *my own outcome*. You should only be interested in your outcome!

If you have been diagnosed with a condition or with a cancer, you should only be interested in the dis-ease or the form of cancer that *you* are living with at this moment. General statistics are meaningless because we are not statistics, averages, or conditions; we are living people who choose to be involved in the outcome of our health. To have a say-so in our health, **WE**––not a doctor–– **need to take charge of our health care**. Taking charge of what happens to us helps us avoid becoming just another statistic, body, case, or number on the protocol-driven conveyor belt of today's healthcare system.

Viktor Frankl, M.D., psychiatrist, holocaust and concentration camp survivor, wrote in his book, *Man's Search For Meaning,* in regard to survival: *"With the loss of belief in the future he* [another inmate] *also lost his spiritual hold. He let himself decline and become subject to physical and mental decay."* (**Note:** The original title of his book translated from German is, *Nevertheless, Say 'Yes' to Life.* That's good advice!)

With cancer (or any other immune system condition), you may have noticed an interesting phenomenon that occurs when one speaks to authorities in the conventional medical field about this or any other life-threatening condition: The more generally you inquire about a condition, the more specific the "authorities" answers seem to be. And the more specific your questions are (i.e., about you or me), the more general the answers become.

Kind of frustrating, isn't it? Please know that I do not expect this book to give you *THE* answer. However, I hope to give you other options, resources, and alternatives to chemotherapy, drugs, radiation, and surgery. Knowing that you have alternatives and other options allows you the opportunity to be in charge of your health care, and possibly have a longer and healthier life. Most importantly, I hope this book will encourage you to take charge of your life and your health, so that you can enjoy however many years or decades you have left to live. You will determine, choose, and find *YOUR* answers.

If you have been diagnosed with melanoma, you probably have been told that you have one to five years to live, or possibly as little as six months. Statistically speaking, approximately 70 percent of individuals diagnosed with melanoma do not live past five years from the time of diagnosis. (2)

Many who have been diagnosed with most other forms of cancer and follow the traditional chemotherapy and radiation protocols have a heightened risk of dying of a heart attack, stroke or another cancer decades later -- a risk that is likely to be due to the original treatment.(3)

The bottom line is, even if you have not been diagnosed with a life-threatening condition, none of us are getting out of this life alive. To put it another way, *life is a fatal disease.* This book is about helping you *live your best life possible, for as many years as possible.* It really is about "you" and not cancer, or any other condition.

3 THOUGHTS FOR YOU TO CONSIDER

The best way to predict the future is to create it. – Peter Drucker

Before reading further, I'd like you to take a moment and answer some questions. As you answer, pay close attention to the first answers that come to your mind because they can be very insightful. Write down your answers on a separate piece of paper so you can refer to them easily. And remember, there are no right or wrong answers; this is not a pass or fail.

1. What does the diagnosis you have been given mean to you?
2. What are you afraid of?
3. What does your diagnosis keep you from doing (in all areas of your life)?
4. What do you want to do in your lifetime? (Dream big! Think short-term, long-term, family, vocation, avocation, etc.)
5. What are your life-guiding values?
6. What is most important to you?

In order to restore your health, it is important that your actions are in alignment with *what you want your life to be*, not what somebody else wants, desires, or needs your life to be. If you answer these questions honestly, they'll help you prioritize your next steps. Also, answering these questions can help you better commit to the necessary actions you need to take for the rest of your life, leading to a more fulfilled, healthier, and satisfied life for you (and secondarily, for those around you).

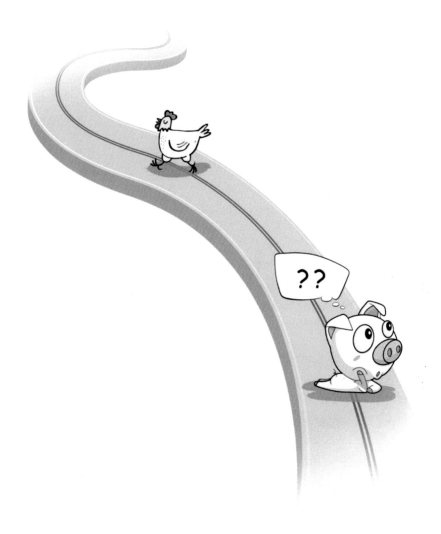

4 YOU HAVE CHOICES

If you can see your path clearly laid out before you, it's not your path.
– David Whyte

Before you can make good health care choices, it is important to first understand how our conventional healthcare system functions. To do this, I would like to share a short story/analogy that demonstrates the relationship between you and any doctor or health care provider, whether conventional or alternative:

> A chicken and a pig were walking down the road when they came upon a restaurant with a sign that read, Bacon & Eggs - $1.95. The chicken turned to the pig and said, "Let's have some breakfast." The pig looked at the chicken and replied, "Let me think about this for a moment." Looking puzzled, the chicken asked, "Why?" The pig replied, "For you, this breakfast is just a donation; for me, it is total commitment."
> The doctor is the chicken, and you are the pig.

Understand that the vast majority of providers, both conventional and alternative, are truly dedicated to helping you to restore your health and regain your life; however, all providers are "chickens" and can only make "donations." How you choose to respond to the diagnosis you have received and the decisions you make is "total commitment". You are the one who may pay for those decisions with your life.

I suggest that you relate this little story to your doctor(s) to help them understand that you want to be in charge of your health. It can give them insight into the role you see them playing in your health care, and give them notice that you are more than a "warm body" for them to treat. It might even be helpful to see how a doctor reacts to determine if this is the person who you want assisting you in your return to health.

Now, with the above analogy in mind, you have some choices to make. First, ask yourself:

Am I going to be an object to be treated, a statistic,
or am I going to be in charge of my life and be proactive in changing my life?

Inside of this decision, there are additional choices that you must make as you wind your way through the maze of health care (or sickness care) options.

A few of the fundamental decisions you'll be making are:

- Conventional medicine, alternative health care, or a combination of both
- Good quality of life vs. a possible extension of life (with a possible lower quality of life)
- Helpless vs. "taking charge"
- Disease vs. best possible adaptation

In making these decisions, it is important that you first understand a few things about health and healing. Understand that *cancer* is a generic term for an uncontrolled proliferation of abnormal cells. Inside the alternative vitalist perspective, this proliferation in reality is not wrong, bad, or unnatural. What we call *cancer*, an *autoimmune disease*, or any other condition is a natural (albeit unwanted) response to our internal and external environments. It is a response to a mental, physical, and/or chemical environment that may have began when we were a fetus. Inside the conventional medical perspective, these conditions indicate that the genes and/or cells are broken and need to be fixed. At various times, both of these perspectives can be valid, and we will look into some of the differences between the two later on.

The current medical––allopathic, reductionist, or atomist––approach is to identify, fight, resist, and destroy abnormal cells and harmful organisms, and to reduce and suppress symptoms of the disease. It is important to understand that cancer and most other immune conditions are not diseases; instead, they are *syndromes* (i.e., a group of symptoms). These groups of symptoms, with few exceptions, have no known common causes other than the person's *environment*, and that will vary from person to person. Some researchers feel that attempting to destroy cancer cells with chemotherapy or radiation might cause an increase of up to 350 percent in cancer cell activity. (4) These unwanted cells are attempting to survive. Additionally, some doctors are of the opinion that many patients who have been treated with chemotherapy and/or radiation will not be alive 10 years later, as they will have succumbed to a more vigorous return of the original cancer, or a different form of cancer. (For example, the potential for developing leukemia increases after radiation.)

These unwanted conditions are in response to living in a toxic environment, one that triggers a genetic response resulting in a proliferation of abnormal cells and/or altered immune responses. In the majority of circumstances, your genes are a "potential" and not an absolute or inevitable predictor of any condition. Genes respond to their environment. They don't suddenly go crazy or just stop working without a reason. Yes, certain genes can predispose a person to a condition; however, as noted earlier, they are *potential and not, in most cases, inevitable* predeterminations. Cancer cells, as with all cells, have within them the same programming for survival as we do. Fighting against and trying to destroy these cells creates within them a survival, fight or flight response mechanism as they attempt to continue to live.

It has been estimated that of the millions of new cells your body produces every day, 1 percent are potentially malignant cancer, and your body disposes of these cells quite readily. Your body is programmed to protect, repair, and heal itself, "IF" we provide it with the proper tools.

Cancer, dis-ease, or a sickness is like luck; it occurs at the intersection of preparation and opportunity.

How you eat and exercise, the chemicals you have been exposed to (prenatal and postnatal), and your mental/emotional state, whether you are aware of it or not, produced an environment that became toxic and conducive to whatever state of dis-ease you may be experiencing today.

Understand that for the best possible outcome, your focus in regard to any of these conditions must be on strengthening your ability to be healthy. Focusing on the disease magnifies the condition. That keeps you from living your life. Resisting the condition––instead of building up your body's health and resistance––takes your attention away from your long-term goal of living a healthy and happy life. This is not to say that you should deny the condition; instead, put it in its proper place and perspective in your life.

Within the "trains" metaphor, a mental visual that helped me was thinking of melanoma as an unwanted and unexpected boxcar that was added to my "train," or that my life was on one set of tracks, and melanoma was temporarily on a parallel set of tracks. The tracks could converge and the trains could crash, or my train (or the other train) could be diverted in another direction. All of these visuals helped me to hold onto my life, and put the condition in its proper context, relative to my life.

When you identify with the cancer, or any condition, by resisting or taking personal possession of it––by using terms like *my cancer*, or *I have* breast cancer, *I have* skin cancer, or *I have* fibromyalgia, or whatever it might be––you are in essence giving the dis-ease syndrome an identity and personality. Also, believing that dis-ease must be *driven out, killed, or removed,* gives it a personality; it gives existence to the condition. I prefer to say, *I was diagnosed with a melanoma.* (I suggest you do the same with whatever your condition might be.) I do not identify with melanoma or personalize this adaptation to my previous environment beyond the code name that identifies a set of symptoms or tissues involved. I have not allowed it to become who I am or my life. *Remember, you and I are not our dis-eases!* This is not to say that we should live in a state of denial of our circumstances. Malignant melanoma, cancers, and other dis-eases are real responses to what is happening in our bodies, and they require real actions on our part; however, anything we resist, fight, or oppose, will always gain strength from our resistance.

Example of Strength from Resistance: Ask someone to extend their arm toward you with their palm facing you, and give no further instruction. Now, take your hand and push against their palm. They will almost always automatically push back against your hand. To resist pressure is a normal instinctual response that is built into all living structures, down to the microscopic level.

Look at trees that must constantly fight strong winds; they are stronger.

And the butterfly must work against the "resistance" of the chrysalis or cocoon to strengthen their wings to be able to fly.

"Focusing on" cancer or any condition gives it an identity, and "resisting" a dis-ease gives it more strength and life. Rather than worrying about or fearing the dis-ease, it is important to understand why this dis-ease is present in the first place. The goal is not to feel guilty or blame anyone, but to better understand. With this knowledge we can strengthen our bodies to alter the malignant response to our previous environment the dis-ease represents.

Trees cannot change their environment.

The Butterfly needs the chrysalis to be able to fly and to survive.

You are not a tree or a butterfly.

You don't need cancer, and you can change your environments.

Understand, accept, and change would be my suggestion.

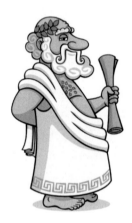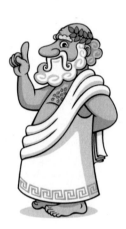

5 A LITTLE HISTORY

The good physician treats the disease; the great physician treats the patient who has the disease. – Sir William Osler

It may help to understand that today's medical model is based on a premise that was championed by Democritus 2500 years ago when he debated Hippocrates. (In reality, Hippocrates is the father of what we today call *alternative medicine*; not conventional medicine, as many incorrectly believe.) Hippocrates argued that there was an inherent power in the body that self-regulates and works to maintain the body in a state of health or balance (i.e., homeostasis). Democritus countered that Hippocrates was espousing religion, and that only through scientific understanding of the body's physical makeup could health be maintained. Later, Benjamin Rush, M.D. (also a signer of the Declaration of Independence), expanded on Democritus' position with the comment, "It is the "art" of the physician to take the role of healing out of nature's hands." (5)

Today's conventional medical model of health care is *reductionist*; looking for the primary, most basic fundamental structures and entities––chemical, genetic, viral and/or bacterial––that could be the cause of a malady or dis-ease. It addresses the symptoms of a condition and the end stage of dis-ease. This paradigm generally views the body as a group of loosely connected parts, housed in a "skin bag," unable to fully function or survive for long without outside intervention. This perspective generally sees the body as susceptible to breaking down or being invaded by outside influences, and unable to defend or repair itself without assistance. It holds that the body is equal to or less than, the sum of its

17

parts, removing the person and life from the equation. This does not mean that the conventional physician does not care about the individual. Their methods and interventions, however, require them to disassociate from the patient in order to treat and focus on the "dis-ease" entity, symptoms, or effects.

The underlying premise behind most alternative health care is *vitalism*. The vitalist position holds that the body is made up of many interrelated and interactive parts, and that the whole is greater than the sum of its parts. The vitalist acknowledges the inherent healing ability of the body as they work with that innate ability to help it heal (or adapt), to return the body to a state of homeostasis (balance). Inside of this paradigm, the dis-ease is the result of the body adapting to the environment its been exposed to––chemically, physically, emotionally, nutritionally, and to a limited extent, genetically. The intention of the vitalist approach is to help the patient change toxic and harmful factors in their environment or lifestyle to allow the body to return to optimal function. This is not to deny the need for conventional medical intervention in life-threatening events; however, these medical interventions should be considered temporary, to be supported by nutritional, emotional, and physical interventions in order for the body to heal and compensate from the damage that drugs and surgery will create. It requires that the individual be informed about as many factors impacting their health as possible, and that they actively participate in their own return to health. From the vitalist perspective the person is in charge of their own recovery, not a helpless victim to be saved.

Briefly summarized, the conventional paradigm holds that the body is dysfunctional, it has been invaded, or it is missing something, and that it is necessary to replace, modify, or remove some *unnecessary* parts, or to remove or kill an invading organism before the body can return to non-impaired function. The alternative vitalist approach holds that the body is whole, complete, and more than just the sum of its parts, and that it just needs to be strengthened and supported to function properly.

The conventional approach strives to *prevent death*; the vitalist approach strives to *promote health*. The conventional approach looks for *the what*; the vitalist looks for *the why*. Both of these paradigms are valid and appropriate at various times, and they are not mutually exclusive. In other words, they can be used to complement each other for the benefit of your good health.

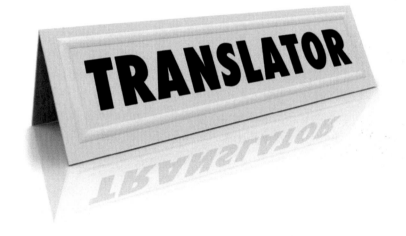

6 UNDERSTANDING TERMINOLOGY

You keep using that word. I do not think it means what you think it means.

– Inigo, from The Princess Bride

The above quote is one of my favorites from one of my favorite movies, and it captures our dilemma when it comes to communication between a doctor and a patient (the chicken and pig). Understanding terminology gives you more knowledge about the therapies, medications, and procedures that are being recommended. Understanding terminology in regard to the outcomes and goals that you and your doctor discuss (and how they might differ), places you on the same team and pulling in the same direction as your doctor. Be sure that you understand the terminology being used by your doctor and other healthcare providers.

Below is a list of key terms that I think you should know. The list is not all-inclusive, but it's a good place to start when raising questions about your health care:

> **Cure** – Your cure is up to you. No drug, surgery, or intervention can *cure* you. Interventions can give your body the opportunity it needs to restore itself to a healthier state, but they do not *cure* the types of conditions we are talking about. You must change your lifestyle and the environment your body is in before you can expect a *cure* and/or to have a healthier and longer lifespan. And in order to be *cured,* you must continue those lifestyle changes until you don't want to be *cured* any

longer. In other words, there is no *cure*; there is only a change in the environment or circumstances that can result in a healthier outcome.

Questions to Ask Your Doctor: "Doctor, what is your definition of *cure*?"

Dis-ease – Having a lack of ease, a state of imbalance, unhealthy function, or unhealthy response. Think of *dis-ease* as a deviation from that which otherwise would be healthy or optimal function.

Questions to Ask You Doctor: "Doctor, can you explain why I have this condition?" "What is the underlying cause of this condition?" Note whether his answer makes sense to you or is unclear or ambiguous.

Effective – A term used to indicate that the applied therapy created the intended result, i.e., *it is effective in lowering the mortality rate*, or *one plus one equals two*. With cancer, this could mean that the therapy caused cancer cells to die, since that is the desired result. However, please note that the statements of effectiveness speak solely to whether or not the treatment produced a desired result. We do not know if the treatment produced the true end result *we* had *hoped for*. Important considerations can remain unaddressed, like...*without causing reduced quality of life or life expectancy*. Questions like, *for how long and at what physical cost*, need to be addressed. In summary, if the doctor is saying that the therapy is effective, you need to understand what exactly they mean by *effective*? Are they telling you that the therapy has efficacy and they think that the therapy will work for *YOU*? Know *exactly* what effect the doctor is expecting. It may not include the *effects* you wanted or that you thought he meant.

Questions to Ask Your Doctor: "Doctor, what do you mean by *effective*?" "For how long was it effective in the studies, and to what extent?" "Did this (therapy/drug/procedure) eliminate, reduce, or modify the condition I am asking you to help me with?" "What side effects are associated with this therapy?"

Efficacy – A term that is used to validate a concept or theory. For example, *it worked in laboratory studies and in theory, but we aren't sure how effective it is*, or *it causes a response of some kind that we think will cause the desired outcome*. In other words, we think this will work, let's try it out and see. It is like flu inoculations; it creates an increase in antibody production in humans, so there is *efficacy*. However, it is not *effective* in changing the mortality rate or in lowering the incidence of the flu. (6) In addressing chronic conditions and cancer syndromes, there are many therapies that have efficacy but may not be effective for everyone, or as effective as other alternatives, or they do not produce the results we expect.

<u>Questions to Ask Your Doctor</u>: "Doctor, has this (therapy/treatment/drug) been shown to reduce, affect, or eliminate this particular condition, and if so, to what extent?" "Can you provide me with the actual numbers?"

Functional Medicine (FM) – You will probably not hear this term while under conventional medical care; however, it is one that you should become familiar with. *Functional medicine* looks at the patient from a functional and vitalistic perspective, as a *person*; not from a sickness perspective, as a *disease*. Your FM practitioner could be a D.C. (Doctor of Chiropractic), an M.D. (Medical Doctor), a D.O. (Doctor of Osteopathy), a N.D. (Doctor of Naturopathy), an A.R.N.P. (Advanced Registered Nurse Practitioner), or a P.A. (Physicians Assistant). They use laboratory and physical testing, similar to what a conventional practitioner would use; however, they look for clinical and sub-clinical signs of dysfunction. They also look at a collection of symptoms, signs, and findings that may define a syndrome (rather than a single cause of a disease). Additionally, they will also look at the person's diet, lifestyle, occupation and emotional status that may be contributing to the disease.

The FM practitioner looks at multiple organs, glands, systems, and functions, in an attempt to integrate various clinical and laboratory findings. They seek to address the unique underlying cause of deficiency in each patient, individually. Simply put, the FM doctor is concerned with *the why* of a condition, as opposed to conventional medicine's focus on *the what*. I am telling you this now because you may want to consider consulting this type of practitioner to assist you in returning to good health.

Goals – These are the outcomes we desire. Be sure to make your goals clear to every health care provider you have when seeking treatment.

Often, the doctor's goal will be to kill cancer cells, when your goal is to live a longer life and have a good quality of life. (Your goal is whatever it is that *you* define it to be.) This brings to mind the old cliché, *the operation was a success, but the patient died.* Always be clear when expressing your goals for the outcome that you want from the treatment that your health care provider is suggesting to you. After their suggested treatment, do you want to be alive, cancer free, have a good quality of life, a normal life span, no cancer return, not to be disabled, etc.?

Be sure to have a clear understanding of what your practitioner's goals are, what their definition of *success* is, and what measures they are using to define that *success*. (For me, a 7 percent chance of gaining five extra months at the price of having the flu for a year was not an optimistic goal, but you might feel differently.)

Questions to Ask Your Doctor: "Doctor, my goals from your treatments are (_____). What are your goals for me from your treatments?" "In your opinion, are my goals realistic?"

Health – The World Health Organization defines health as; *health is a state of complete physical, mental, and social wellbeing, and not merely the absence of disease or injury.* Health, simply put, is your body in a state of optimal function.

Questions to Ask Your Doctor: "Doctor, what is your primary goal; to get rid of my symptoms (i.e., cancer) or to improve my health?" If they reply, "Both", then ask, "Which is most important to you, Doctor?"

Life Expectancy – Based on similar cases, this is the medical *average* of how long a person is expected to survive after diagnosis. (Notice that the key word here is *average*.) Decide to exceed expectations and to be above average!

Questions to Ask Your Doctor: "Doctor, how long can I expect to live with your treatment, and how long without it?" "Will you provide me with the actual numbers and references to support your suggested treatment?"

Number Needed to Treat (NNT) – You may not have heard of this term before, but it is one that you should become familiar with. Therapies, drugs, and interventions are not effective for everyone. NNT asks the question, *how many people out of how many people* *had the intended outcome?* (In other words, is the treatment worth considering?)

*EXAMPLE: Statin medications are noted to be effective in reducing the incidence of heart events by 50 percent. This sounds good; however, what is not being said is that in this study, on average, approximately 100 participants (reportedly) needed to treat in order to prevent only one more heart attack vs. the placebo. So your odds are 1 in 100 that it will help. (7) (****Note:*** No mention was made of how many people will experience a variety of side effects from this medication.)*

<u>Questions to Ask Your Doctor</u>: "Doctor, from the therapy you are recommending, how many people with my condition had a good outcome, what do you qualify as a good outcome, and how many people were treated with the therapy you are recommending?"

Outcomes – When doctors speak of successful outcomes, be sure to ask them what they mean. The literature may note that the treatment had a successful outcome because a therapy increased the *average,* predicted lifespan for someone with that disease by a few months. This is similar to making a prognosis, and it applies to procedures, therapies, and syndromes. Be sure that the outcome the doctor is speaking of is one you desire and is acceptable to you. (Ag*ain, we don't want a successful surgical or chemical outcome, but the patient died a horrible death.*) Ask yourself, from *whose perspective* is the outcome considered successful, and what measures of success are being utilized?

<u>Questions to Ask You Doctor</u>: "Doctor, what outcome are you expecting from this therapy, and what are the potential physical and emotional costs to me?" "Is this a permanent or temporary (short-term) outcome?"

Percentages – Often, a doctor will say that a medication or procedure reduced a symptom or the mortality rate by some percentage rate like 50%. You may interpret this as okay odds; however, when we look deeper into the statin study (mentioned earlier) we see it was a double-blind study where 8,900 of the participants took a statin medication, and 8,900 participants took a placebo. 2.8 percent (251) of the participants who did not take the medication had heart events over the course of the study, and out of the group who took the medication, 1.6 percent (142 participants) had a heart event.

Thus, statin was shown to be 50 percent more effective than the placebo. (**Note**: It took 8,900 people to get these numbers, and adverse reactions to the medication were not discussed.) (7) The lesson here is, don't be taken in by percentages; instead, ask your provider for real numbers, for example, the number of people that needed to be treated to obtain those numbers.

Questions to Ask Your Doctor: "Doctor, what are the *actual numbers* of people treated and those who recovered, compared to those who were given a placebo or were in non-treated controls?"

Publication Bias – *(As noted previously, given my experiences, I have a bias for alternative, vitalistic, natural care and therapy, and I am skeptical of traditional medical practices.)*

When reading published papers, blogs, books, and online content (and even when speaking with doctors), be aware of any bias or prejudice that the author, publisher, or doctor may have. Ask yourself, was the author attempting to prove a personal opinion of theirs? Did a pharmaceutical or supplement company who will profit from the findings fund the study? Is the author directly or indirectly profiting from the favorable comments regarding a therapy or a remedy? Did a specific company fund the researcher, and is this disclosed? Are all the results, both good and bad, reported, or are only the favorable ones to the author's point of view reported? In what is called a *meta-analysis* (a review of published papers searching for patterns) did the research include unpublished and/or contrary papers? Not all research is created equal, and humans (with human frailties) are the ones who are doing the research. It has been estimated that up to 50 percent of all material published today has some degree of publication bias, ranging from minor human error, to out-and-out fraud. (9)(10)

Questions to Ask Your Doctor: "Doctor, if you were in my shoes, would you take this medication/have this surgery?" "Doctor, other than being paid for your service, are there any other personal, financial, educational, or emotional considerations that are going into your recommendations to me?"

> *When schemes are laid in advance, it is surprising how often the circumstances will fit in with them.*
>
> – Sir William Osler, a founder of John Hopkins Hospital

Prognosis – Similar to life expectancy, this is a medical determination for the duration or course of a dis-ease It is the ultimate outcome of a dis-ease; a verbal picture of what your doctor expects will happen, based on the literature and the experience of the doctor. It is not a "given" for any one person in any one case; instead, it is an educated guess. (Remember, if you are reading this, you are not a statistic yet!)

Questions to Ask Your Doctor: "Doctor, what do you foresee as the course of my life, having this condition?"

Quality of Life – This is a prognosis of your level of comfort, ability to function, move, and be active, addressing the type of life that you will be able to have. You are the one who must consciously decide what is acceptable for you.

Questions to Ask Your Doctor: "Doctor, what will be my quality of life if I take your treatment, and what quality of life will I have if I don't?"

Response Rate – This is a term typically used with percentages. It is important that you know the NNT (Number Needed to Treat) and what is meant by *response rate*. When they say, *response*, was it a total remission or a rash? Is the *response* you thought they were talking about a cure, an increase in your lifespan, an improvement to your quality of life (and by how much), or was it an *academic response* (cells were killed, a rash was seen, antibodies were formed, etc.)

Questions to Ask Your Doctor: "Doctor, what do you mean by *response*, and how many people had this response out of how many people in the trial?" "For how long did they have it, and what were the side effects when they did?"

Remission – Simply put, remission means that there is no further evidence of the dis-ease, condition, or syndrome; however, it may re-occur. No one can say for sure when it might reoccur, or if it will. Lifestyle syndromes are never really cured. Instead, they enter into an indefinite state of remission. Typically, the duration depends on the patient's willingness to alter their eating, thinking, and moving habits.

Questions to Ask Your Doctor: "Doctor, by *remission,* does that mean the condition is cured, or do you mean that the condition is temporarily on hold?" "If on hold, for how long is it on hold?"

Syndrome – A syndrome is a collection of symptoms and findings that do not have a single, identifiable cause. Cancer, fibromyalgia, autoimmune conditions, etc., are all syndromes that do not have a single, identifiable cause (other than *lifestyle*).

Questions to Ask Your Doctor: "Doctor, what do you believe has caused this condition?"

Remember when discussing your health with your healthcare provider do not be afraid to ask, what does that mean? What do you mean by that? Can you explain in simple terms so I can understand? Can I see the studies supporting your recommendation? Do not assume anything. This is not the time to be shy or worry about what someone else will think of you! Understand that doctors are human beings, too. They don't like telling people bad news; they like being right, and want to be liked. Remember too, that sometimes *what you think you hear* may not be what was said.

And never be afraid to seek out a second (or third, or more) opinion.

Suggestion: Any time you see a doctor, write out your questions and concerns, and bring them with you to your visit. If possible, have someone go with you to help you remember to ask all of your questions. They can also help you remember the doctor's answers after you've left the office.

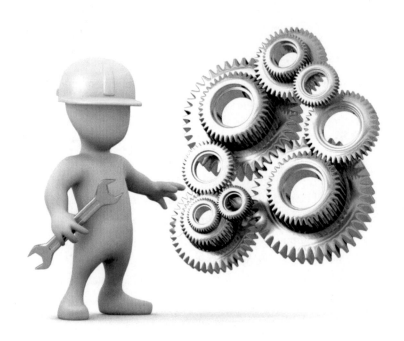

7 THE MEDICAL MODEL

The art of medicine consists in amusing the patient, while
nature cures the disease. – Voltaire

Conventional medicine has basically four methods for treating cancer and other conditions: surgery, immune/metabolic therapies, chemotherapy/drugs, and/or radiation. This medical model attacks the cancer and/or the symptom. Simplistically speaking, conventional physicians are trained to look for and identify invading organisms, diseased cells, and/or abnormally functioning organs in order to kill, replace, suppress, or remove the offending organisms, organs, cells, and/or symptoms. This approach is appropriate when faced with immediate life or death circumstances and in a few other situations like reconstructive surgery, temporary pain relief or to repair the result of accident or injury. However, no surgery or medication is free of side effects or unintended consequences. You must first clearly understand the intended result of any procedure, and be informed of any potential ill side effects you might experience as a result of that procedure.

In an editorial I read a few years ago, in the online medical news publication, *The American Medical News,* it stated that the working, yet, unacknowledged, philosophy of medicine was based on the theory that, *"The elimination of all sickness and disease will leave you with health."* When viewed in the light of day, it's easy to see that this philosophy is flawed and untrue. Unfortunately, it is apparent that this philosophy remains the obvious unstated philosophy that many conventional providers align themselves with despite the lack of logic behind it. This is neither good nor bad; however, it is something you need to be aware of when dealing with our conventional healthcare system.

Your doctor and every other healthcare provider that you see should be viewed as a coach, consultant, source of information, and/or highly trained technician (a chicken) who you hired to help discover your options, decide on your plan of action, and to provide technical expertise *after YOU* (the pig) decide on a course of action. You should be made aware of all of your doctor's biases and knowledge limitations, and because you will be the one living with the results of any action taken, you also need to *be aware of all of your available alternatives,* even if the provider does not believe in, accept, or endorse those therapies. This is called *informed consent.*

For me, considering that it was malignant melanoma and where the melanoma was located, removing the lesion made sense to me; however, every case––whether melanoma or some other form of cancer or condition––is unique. It is up to you to weigh the benefits vs. the residual side effects of any surgery or medication. Some medical authorities are of the opinion that surgically removing the lesion on my shoulder would cause it to metastasize more rapidly. However, I felt that removing the lesion was the best path, given my (not necessarily your) circumstances, and the location of the lesion. Today, three-and-a-half years and four surgeries later, I am missing a quarter of my left trapezius muscle, half of the lymph nodes under my left arm, and I lack the ability to fully abduct––lift away from my body––my arm over my head (although for me at this point in time, that is a minor inconvenience). As this is being written, I'm told that *medically,* I'm cancer free. This surgery has given me a chance to change my life, and to change my internal and external environments so that cancer cells can no longer survive.

In cancer syndromes, odds and outcomes after conventional therapy are not overly optimistic. Radiation and chemotherapy have been shown to have varying degrees of success with a few types of cancer; however, there are few conventional therapies that provide for a normal life span.

In the following section, I briefly address each of the five standard, conventional medical therapies used to treat cancer syndromes and other immune conditions. My intent is to give you more information in regard to which therapies to utilize, and to make you aware of some of the limitations of these therapies, as well.

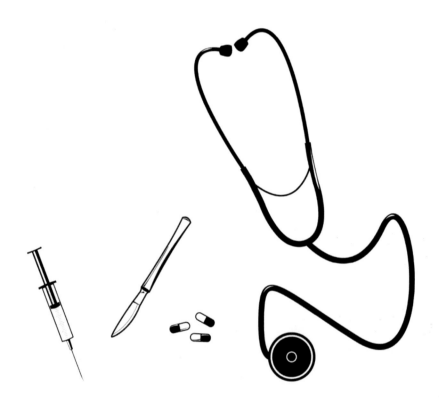

8 CONVENTIONAL MEDICAL THERAPIES

Medicine in higher health acts as an enabler of irresponsibility.
– Deepak Chopra, M.D.

Surgery: For many with early stage and localized cancer syndromes, surgery can be an attractive option. It removes the involved tissue, and depending on the site of the lesion, it can have minimal, long-term ill-effects. However, some authorities believe that by surgically disturbing the lesion and tissue, we could be giving the malignant cells easier access to the bloodstream, causing it to metastasize. There are no studies to support this logic, but it is something to consider. Surgery also lowers your body's resistance and weakens your immune system, making you more susceptible to additional opportunistic organisms. Surgery creates a significant insult to the body because it invades areas that were never intended be exposed to external influences. However on the positive side, surgery can remove a massive section of the tissue in question that posed an immediate threat to your body.

You will note that I mention above that I am missing "half of the lymph nodes under my left arm." In treating cancer surgically, standard procedure, when regional lymph nodes are involved, is to remove all the lymph nodes in that area. I refused to allow this to be done to me. I insisted that the surgeon remove only those nodes that he thought were cancerous and healthy nodes were to be left in place. Lymph nodes are filters, they are an essential part of the immune system and I wanted those filters left in place. By leaving the healthy nodes in place they can continue to prevent further spread or metastasis of the cancer and the immune system still has the benefit of these tissues in producing the white blood cells known as lymphocytes. An additional concern, besides removing an important aspect of the immune system, is that removing all the lymph nodes leaves one susceptible to what is known as lymphedema. Lymphedema occurs after destruction of lymph nodes causing the possibility of fluid accumulating in the affected arm or leg. This accumulation in turn then can lead to infection and gangrene and possibly the loss of the limb. I strongly suggest that you have a serious talk with your surgeon about leaving healthy lymph nodes in place if they are recommending removal of any lymph nodes.

In conclusion, surgery can be a logical option for improving your chances of having a good long-term outcome in a variety of instances when there are solid tumors. If you choose to have surgery, however, you need to strengthen your body before and after in order to recover more rapidly. For example, it's important to increase the amount of anti-inflammatory herbs and supplements you take, and to include five to ten hyperbaric oxygen therapy sessions before and after surgery to help accelerate your healing process, your recovery and to help the surgery be more effective.

> If you have decided to have surgery, I strongly recommend that you have hyperbaric oxygen therapy before and after surgery. Five to ten sessions can speed up the healing process and repair of any surgically damaged tissue. (This is in addition to taking nutritional supplements and nutrients before and after surgery to help you heal faster, as well.)

Chemotherapy: Chemotherapy utilizes toxic poisons intended to kill cancer cells. It is, however, an indiscriminate therapy––a poison––that kills healthy cells along with malignant cells. In other words, chemotherapy is a race to see who will die first. *Will it be you or the cancer?* In many cases not all cancer cells are killed. Some malignant cells survive because they were less affected by the therapy. They can become genetically adapted to the chemical toxins from the chemotherapy (gene amplification) and now can better resist these toxic chemicals the second time chemotherapy is administered. (11) This process, when accompanied by a weakened immune system, is why in the majority of cases, a return cancer is more aggressive and resistant to therapy after the second diagnosis. Because of this increased resistance, and the toll it takes on the body, it is even more important at this point to change your lifestyle, and build your strength and immune system should you opt to have chemotherapy in the future.

Many are under the impression that chemotherapy cures cancer syndromes after a few days or weeks of taking some drug, but nothing could be further from the truth. In most cases, chemotherapy is an uncomfortable inpatient/outpatient intravenous therapy that takes hours to administer, multiple times a week, over the course of several months. These potent drugs weaken the immune system, making you more susceptible to infection and secondary cancers. Brain fog, fatigue, flu-like symptoms, a weakened heart, vomiting, nerve damage and hair loss are just a few of the unpleasant side effects of chemotherapy. These side effects can extend indefinitely, even after the therapy has been discontinued.

This method of therapy typically includes multiple combinations of potent medications in hope that one will work. Combining these drugs together increases the unexpected side effects that can occur when administered. The bottom line is, chemotherapy treatments are no walk in the park. It has been, however, shown to be of long-term benefit when treating a few forms of cancer. This is something that should be considered in the context of quality vs. quantity of life. In other words, ask yourself if the outcome is good enough for you to warrant the pain, cost, and possible disability you might need to endure for the length of time that you would have to endure it.

NOTE: In 2004, the medical journal, *Clinical Oncology,* reported a study that showed with few exceptions, chemotherapy treatments had an impact of only 2.1 percent on the five-year survival rates in the United States. (12)

It should also be noted that when surveyed, 75 percent of the 118 doctors involved in cancer treatment and research at McGill University said they would not have chemotherapy treatments if diagnosed with some form of cancer. (13)

Immunotherapy: The third approach taken by conventional medicine is *immunotherapy*. This therapy is similar to chemotherapy, in that it is applied through intravenous injections. Like chemotherapy, immunotherapy can have multiple, unpleasant side effects. Immunotherapy utilizes cells from the involved cancer syndrome tissue and it attempts to create antibodies to destroy the abnormal cells. This is a relatively new therapy with some degree of promise, as it attempts to use the body to alter the condition. All these therapies are still in the testing stages, however, with limited success. For example, with YERVOY® (generic ipilimumab, the drug for advanced inoperable melanoma), a ten-month survival rate is considered a good outcome. However, it has resulted in positive outcomes for only a small number of patients, at a significant financial cost, and the success comes with the need to endure the many side effects of this therapy.

Radiation: Radiation is the fourth tool that conventional medicine uses to treat cancer syndromes. Radiation is effective in killing malignant cancer cells (and healthy cells). Radiation is as indiscriminate as chemotherapy, and like chemotherapy, radiation is not a therapy that you can narrow down to only the malignant lesion in question. Granted, in one respect it is more focused than chemotherapy; however, radiation has a systemic impact and local effects that can often result in a variety of new cancers and/or leukemia. Additionally, radiation suppresses the immune system (creating increased malignant cell resistance factors, as I mentioned earlier). Also, it is important to note that tissues burned by radiation do not easily heal. This creates a delay in recovery that can leave the patient susceptible to infection.

In regard to radiation, you should also be aware of the potential damage to tissues surrounding the lesion to be irradiated. You'll want to ask your doctor and surgeon questions like, are there any large nerves or nerve plexuses in close proximity to the lesion? Is the lesion near lung tissue or sensitive organs, like the thyroid? These types of tissues are highly susceptible to damage from radiation. Radiation can cause impaired respiratory function, abnormal hormone production, nerve damage (resulting in nerve impairment), altered metabolism, and reduced respiratory function. Ask questions about these types of tissues if you decide to have radiation therapy.

Pharmaceuticals/Drugs: These are medications for treating syndromes, reducing pain, influencing hormone production, reducing inflammation, and killing viruses and bacteria. All drugs and pharmaceuticals have known side effects when tested individually. But the side effects of two or more medications when prescribed together have *unknown multiple* side effects that can be (and many times are) worse than the dis-ease that they have been prescribed to treat. Remember; medications are prescribed for treating symptoms, suppressing or increasing organ functions, and for killing organisms. They are not prescribed to promote health. If you find it necessary to take a medication, your goal should be to stop taking it within the shortest period of time possible, and to switch to natural alternatives, as soon as possible.

Chemotherapy and radiation are not options that I would consider, but for you, one or both may be a viable option. In some cases--like testicular cancer, lymphoma, and other forms of leukemia--chemotherapy has been shown to have a high rate of success in forcing the cancer into remission for prolonged periods of time (for years, and in some cases, for a lifetime). However, significant doubt must be raised in regard to using these therapies (chemotherapy, biologics, and/or radiation) for other cancers, as the outcomes have been shown to have either limited or marginal success. I also question harm vs. benefit when using these therapies in *a just-to-be-sure-we-got-it-all-after-surgery* mentality, or as part of an overall *protocol* that accompanies surgery. It shouldn't be used *just because.*

When a lesion is small, in its early stage, and is easily accessible, to me it makes sense to remove the lesion. However, the caveat is that you must address and adjust your internal and external environments, and build up your strength and immunity in order to withstand the impact that surgery will have on your body. The same applies if you choose chemotherapy; you must improve your environment and build your body so that cancer or any other condition does not have an opportunity to reoccur and you are strong enough to withstand the toxic effects of the therapy. Improving your lifestyle is always appropriate, either as a means to address the problem or to complement conventional therapies through an integrated approach. Improving your lifestyle will help you become stronger during procedures, as it improves your overall health. Obviously, no matter what therapy or combination of therapies you choose, the goal should be the same––to return to great health, and have the best quality of life possible for the longest period of time possible.

Bottom line, **ASK QUESTIONS** and know the possible consequences of your decisions should you decide to have surgery, take a drug, try immunotherapy, or have radiation. Understand the alternatives that you have available to you for these procedures, as well.

If we were to make an analogy between treating cancer, dis-eases, and war, then surgery, drugs, chemotherapy, radiation, and other conventional therapies could be compared to air bombardment over enemy positions. Bombing is effective as it kills many of the enemy, but there can also be collateral damage to civilians, one's own troops, and community infrastructure. And usually, it will not, in and of itself, cause the enemy to surrender nor can it secure lasting peace. For complete victory you need "feet on the ground" soldiers (i.e., changing your mental, physical, and nutritional habits), and negotiators who can enter the arena and cleanup any remaining enemy, rebuild towns, and restore civilian control or to prevent the occurrence of a war before it starts.

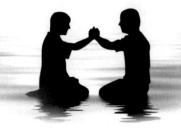

9 VITALIST, ALTERNATIVE OR COMPLEMENTARY

Treat a man as he is, and he will remain as he is. Treat a
man as he could be and he will become what he should be.
– Ralph Waldo Emerson

As noted earlier, the vitalist approach does not focus on the dis-ease; rather, it focuses on the person who has the dis-ease. If you have been diagnosed with a dis-ease, ask yourself questions like, what in my environment is creating this adaptation called "cancer" or other condition? What am I doing that made this dysfunctional set of symptoms––cancer cells, chronic pain, heart conditions, bowel issues, etc.––become an acceptable alternative for what once were healthy cells and systems?

From the vitalist point of view, the body is constantly striving to survive and be healthy for as long as possible. Any malignant, inappropriate, or unhealthy symptoms or tissues are in direct response to the environments we have created, knowingly or not. Much the same as conventional medicine, the alternative provider asks: What is the mental/emotional, physical, chemical, and nutritional history of this individual? What dis-eases, inoculations, injuries, and occupations has this person had? What factors are present or absent that would not be present or absent in a perfectly healthy person? The difference between the vitalist approach and conventional medicine is the doctor's response to these questions. Conventional medicine attempts to address the symptoms; alternative medicine attempts to address the environment that stimulated the symptoms.

The vitalist respects the premise that the body heals, not a drug, doctor, supplement, or potion. (This reminds me of the old saying, the body heals; the physician collects the fee.) This does not mean that conventional interventions are not necessary and appropriate at times; however, it does mean that these interventions should assist the body in its innate and inborn ability to survive and thrive. The difference between the two is perspective and intent. Does the treatment focus on the symptom or the person? Often, both perspectives need to be applied in order to obtain the optimal result. This is known as, complementary medicine or integrative medicine. Once pathological organisms and tissues have been addressed, the environment that created the pathology can now be improved. However, conventional therapies must be re-evaluated relative to the new state of health in the body and its internal environment. At this point, conventional interventions may become more harmful than beneficial, and vitalistic interventions may be needed in order to reestablish homeostasis and restore balance to the body that needs to be strengthened. The prime directive of all healthcare providers is, "First do no harm." The vitalistic model of healthcare is a more ideal paradigm, to provide improved health, and to honor the prime directive.

A fundamental principle of microbiology states, *"The virulence of the disease is inversely proportional to the resistance of the host."* In simple terms this means, the stronger your immune system, the less likely it is that a foreign organism will establish a foothold in your body. Whether they realize it or not, all doctors and healthcare providers work to return you to optimal health. Your immune system must be made strong. The vitalist addresses the whole environment––internal and external––that created the weakening of the immune system in the first place. The vitalist examines **the cause,** and the conventional practitioner attempts to address **the dis-ease or effect** of a weakened immune system.

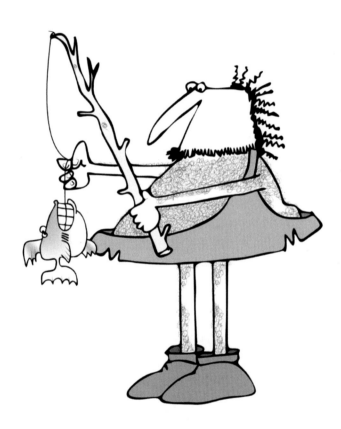

10 A HEALTHY LIFESTYLE

Illness is forgetting wellness.
– Deepak Chopra, M.D.

Loren Cordain, Ph.D. in his book, *The Paleo Diet; Lose Weight and Get Healthy by Eating the Food You Were Designed to Eat,* estimates that genetically, we have not changed but approximately .002 percent in the past 40,000 years. (Be aware that herding and cultivating originated some 10,000 to 20,000 years ago). To me, this creates the perfect template for what should be our level of activity, the foods our bodies need, and the way our bodies respond to our emotional states. In my mind, I can imagine someone following a herd of animals or a fish migration, and setting up camp every other night or so. This person probably eats handfuls of a variety of berries, roots, vegetables, and fruits throughout the day, along with some tasty grubs and insects.

Besides the vegetables and berries, this individual's primary diet most likely consists of eggs, fish, fowl, or herd animal protein in the evening, after the hunt. Then after the evening meal, they relax, sitting around a fire with their family and other tribal members, sharing history, stories, and traditions, which in turn strengthens the bonds within the community and educates the children. For me, this picture is a guide for what to eat and what level of activity I should strive to achieve. (I will pass on the tasty grubs and insects, thank you.) I recommend that everyone read Loren Cordain's book, *The Paleo Diet*, to better understand how our body has evolved to function, when healthy, and how far Western civilization has deviated from this healthy state of living in the last 40,000 years.

In regard to the theory that our genes are the cause for our diminished health, Dr. James Chestnut shares a good analogy in the relationship between genetics, the environment, and dis-ease in many of his presentations. He asks the question, if the fish in the Great Lakes began dying off with cancer and immune diseases, and the eggs of the sea birds around the Great Lakes became too fragile to mature, would your first thought be "these animals all of a sudden had a genetic change," or would you look for possible changes in these creatures' environment? Our genes are not creating our diminished status; our internal and external environments are creating the damage. Working to model our lifestyles as closely as possible to how we were genetically intended to live, eat, exercise, and relax, will give us a much better opportunity to enjoy a longer and healthier life.

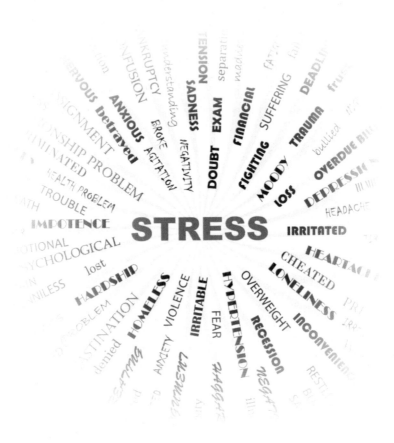

11 HOW DID I GET INTO THIS MESS

I turned my head for a moment, ten years ago, and it became my life.
– David Whyte

Before going into action steps, it is important to know why we need to change our lifestyle. Knowing *the why* will help us understand how our bodies came to produce the syndromes we are experiencing today. Our bodies respond to threats and trauma in similar ways, whether it is physical, emotional, nutritional, or chemical trauma. This response is called a *fight or flight response*, and it physiologically sets into motion an inflammatory response. Think in terms of our Paleolithic man who lived 40,000 years ago. Imagine how his body would respond should he come upon a saber-toothed tiger. First, he'd need to decide if he was going to run or fight. His eyes would dilate; his heart, breathing, and blood pressure would increase; stored sugars would be released; blood flow to his muscles would increase; blood flow to his internal organs would decrease; his bladder and bowel would empty; he would experience short-term memory loss and tunnel vision; his hearing would be reduced; and his insulin resistance, blood clotting function, and cholesterol production would increase.

Sound similar to the lab results we are getting back from our doctors today? Okay, back to our Paleo man...

After his body goes through these changes, he's now prepared to run or fight with a response that's intended to last about 15 minutes, though it could last for longer periods of time. His physical responses would probably last just long enough to run from the tiger, defeat the tiger, or be eaten by the tiger. However, they were never intended to last 16 to 24 hours a day, day in, day out. Also understand that in order for his body to make these systemic adjustments, multiple changes and reactions had to occur in all of the systems in his body––the nervous system; respiratory system; cardiovascular system; digestive/elimination systems; and especially the regulatory organs of his body, including the pituitary gland, thyroid, parathyroid glands, the adrenals, pancreas and the liver–– and they had to be functioning properly. As it was for our Paleo man, it is for us today; all of these reactions have an impact and are a part of our immune system response. Our body works as a unit; an integrated organism of support systems that work together in a concerted effort to maintain, repair, and heal *the whole*. Our bodies are not made up of isolated parts to be removed when one becomes "bad." You cannot have symptoms that are covered up or responses that are suppressed, and expect the body to return to 100 percent health.

The inflammatory response has evolved over literally millions of years and we are creating this response for prolonged periods of time with our modern way of living. The evidence suggests that this is at least partially responsible for what we call today, *diseases of lifestyle*. Heart disease, elevated blood pressure, elevated cholesterol, cancer, fibromyalgia, MS, chronic fatigue, Type II diabetes, irritable bowel syndrome, colitis, autoimmune diseases, and a host of other syndromes, are the result of a prolonged fight or flight inflammatory response. How we eat, think, work, play, rest, our environments, toxic chemical exposures, and the people we surround ourselves with all work together to determine our health. The *dis-ease* is not who we are; instead it's the outcome of how we have been living. Hopefully by now, you are beginning to see how your lifestyle may have created and contributed to your state of health today. Or maybe like me, with melanoma, you can see no clear connect-the-dots pattern as to how you came to this point in your life. Either way, I expect that you are beginning to see that by altering the dysfunctional areas of our lives, we can improve our health and future. However, please do not allow yourself to create guilt over what you may or may not have done in the past. This is no time to beat yourself up over your past. Instead, it is a time to reflect back, note the errors you've made, and make corrections, as best you can.

Also, remember not to allow the symptoms to dictate your life. As I stated earlier, *we are not our condition.* Returning to the "trains" analogy, I like to think of my life, like a freight train, and the melanoma was a boxcar that I mistakenly picked up, that I have now left at a siding. If you are still experiencing the dis-ease, work on finding where the next "siding" is and what you can do in order to leave that "boxcar" on the siding. At the same time, continue to run the train and enjoy the journey.

Again, I cannot repeat often enough how important it is to remember that we are not defined by our diagnosis. **You are not your condition.** You are a person experiencing a number of symptoms that are responses to your environment...period. **This condition is not you!** It is also important to remember, however, that you cannot ignore your situation, as there have been very few miracle spontaneous cures without the person first making changes in their lifestyle. Unless you're in the end stages, left with only weeks or days remaining of a dis-ease, you still have within you the innate ability to change your life and alter the quality of your life for the better. Just remember, *you are in charge* and *you are the cause* (good or bad, whether you want to be or not).

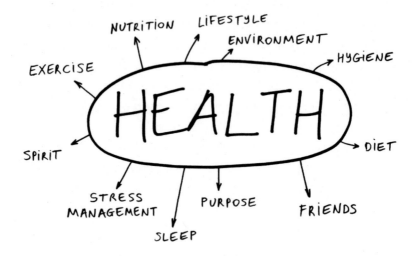

12 AREAS OF HEALTH

Changing health habits out of fear increases the rate of death.

– Deepak Chopra, M.D.

To address the source of trauma in our lives, it is important to be aware of when and how the trauma may have begun. Many theoretical structures have been created to break down the various areas that contribute to our health. Identifying these areas makes it easier to address our strengths, weaknesses and vulnerabilities. For the purposes of this book, I will use a structure that resulted from a dialogue that I participated in that included providers from multiple different health care related disciplines, including conventional medicine, as we explored the topic, *what is health?* This group identified seven interrelated areas of our lives that have an impact on our health today:

1. Physical
2. Mental/Emotional
3. Nutritional/Chemical
4. Environmental
5. Family/Community
6. Occupational
7. Spiritual

(Many in the group also believed that when considering today's modern society, there is an eighth area that also affects our health – Financial.)

I will not delve deeply into each of the seven areas in this book, as it would take me volumes to do so adequately, but hopefully, the following information will help direct you into further investigation of the areas that you need to address.

Physical

Physical trauma is the inflammatory response that is the easiest to avoid and to respond to. It can be due to macro-trauma (like a car accident or fall) or micro-trauma (the result of repetitive motions, poor posture, or bad habits like constantly twisting your neck or back). Physical trauma creates the inflammation that we are most familiar with: redness, swelling, pain, and heat. When tissues are physically traumatized, inflammation occurs around that area and will, depending on the extent of the injury, also activate the immune system in an attempt to protect our vital organs and preserve our lives. Except for repetitive micro-traumas, this is probably the most short-lived cause of inflammation, and the easiest to address because the cause is typically obvious.

In most cases, reducing inflammation that has resulted from physical trauma is best addressed by doing the following: If acute, icing the area for 30 minutes at a time, covering any wounds and keeping the area supple is important. For chronic traumas make sure that your spine is functioning appropriately with spinal adjustments and stretching; exercising (like walking, swimming, and biking) 30-minutes a day in as little as (3) 10-minute sessions this will raise your heart rate, expand your lung capacity, get your blood moving and improve mobility; And, getting between seven to eight hours of restful sleep every night. These are some general actions that will help bring your body back into better function. Just exercising alone for as little as 30 minutes a day will help restore "tone" to the body and can change your world. (**Note:** Once I realized that I did not need to enjoy exercise, and that it was okay to hate the discomfort and time it took, I was able to establish a regular routine.)

Mental/Emotional

It has been my observation that in today's Western society, most emotional stress is the result of *being so busy-being-busy that we have forgotten why we are so busy (if we ever really knew in the first place).* It seems apparent that many people in our society today do not have goals or overarching purposes for their lives beyond what's happening the next weekend. In general, we seem to have only short-term, immediate gratification goals. Having short-term goals inside of intermediate, long-term, and beyond lifetime goals, is sometimes helpful to make the journey through life more manageable and because it helps to maintain a good stress in our lives. Having a sense of over all purpose and meaningful goals is essential to maintaining good health. The journey towards those goals is eased and we are better able to maintain our strength if we are part of a community that supports our goals, ambitions and who we are as a person. And good first steps to reclaiming our peace and direction is having positive practices, like meditation, prayer, a quiet time, and turning off the cell phone, TV, computer, X-box, tablet, and radio to better allow us to focus on what is important in our lives. The mind does not know the difference between real and imagined situations and the body responds to the mind. What are you feeding your mind and how is that causing your body to respond?

Most people think of stress as only bad stress or distress without realizing that there is an alternative. Endocrinologist Dr. Hans Selye used the terms *eustress* and *distress,* and Peter Senge, PhD, American systems scientist and MIT lecturer, uses the terms *creative stress* and *emotional stress.* Bad stress (emotional stress/distress) is fear-based. It can result from having a fear of the future that is based on the past or from guilt over the past. The vast majority of the time, fear is not helpful or healthy. However, good stress, eustress or creative stress, can lead us into action. Good stress causes endorphins to be produced and these neuropeptides help stimulate our immune systems. Good stress excites us, like the anticipation we experience when thinking about vacations and Christmastime. Losing sight of our goals and what's important in life, and only focusing on the things that are wrong, will create emotional or bad stress. Bad stress (fear-based stress) seems to push us away from attaining our goals, while creative or good stress seems to pull us toward those goals. Systematically, good stress stimulates and strengthens the immune system; bad stress suppresses the immune system.

We can enhance our health when we allow ourselves to step back and look at what is important and to plan the next action step in our life. For example, twenty or forty minutes a day of quiet time to just let go and allow ourselves to be at peace, letting our bodies and minds rest, helps us focus and visualize what is truly important in our lives.

A list of goals—a list of things we want to accomplish, do, and/or achieve—gives us purpose and direction. My suggestion would be to make a list of everything that you would like to do before you die and add to it regularly. Your goals don't have to be big, like saving the world or curing cancer. Just having a simple list of things you'd like to accomplish is okay. It's your list; it's no one else's, so list what's important to you. Taking action toward a dream or an exciting goal helps to create healthy responses in your body. Life-threatening and chronic conditions can rob us of our future if we let them and it is important that we don't let them. Take your life back! And if you don't get to accomplish all of your goals, so what? If you have goals, objectives, and dreams, you'll have more fun and enjoy your time on this earth more than if you sit around worrying, whining, and feeling sorry for yourself.

Nutritional/Chemical

What are you eating? Is it real food or plastic food? Is it manufactured and processed with chemicals added? Is it covered in pesticides and inorganic fertilizers? Does it have a label that lists ingredients? Has it been force grown or force fed to produce volume and not nutrition? Is it genetically modified (GMO) or from virgin seeds?

As I mentioned earlier, *The Paleo Diet* is the perfect template for nutrition. It consists of 65 percent organic fruits and vegetables; 35

percent protein from eggs, fish, fowl, and range-fed and range-bled herd animal protein. ("Smoothies" or "juicing" fruits and vegetables is an efficient way to get some of your daily quota) This perfect template avoids grains and dairy in any form. Pragmatically speaking, the goal is have a diet consisting of no more than zero to 20 percent grains. Too many grains can create an inflammatory response in your body. Refined grains and sugars create fat gain and can increase your waist size. Our dependence on grain products is one of our most toxic habits contributing to our lifestyle dis-eases today.

Other major contributors to an inflammatory response are milk and dairy products. Other than mother's milk, milk has a negative impact on our system. As humans, we have not evolved to have dairy in our diets. It is toxic to our bodies and it can create systemic inflammation (clinically and sub-clinically). Therefore, it should be used sparingly, if at all.

Nutritional supplements should never replace whole foods, and they should always be considered a "supplement." However, because of Western civilization's dependence on mass-produced foods from mega-farms, and our addiction to processed foods and plastic foods, it is important to take supplements to ensure we are getting adequate essential nutrients. Taking good supplements is for more than just preventing a deficiency disease. Good supplements can help ensure that your body has adequate nutrition, improves your general health and helps you to resist foreign substances and organisms, as well.

You might notice that the recommendations below exceed the minimum daily requirements, but I prefer to do more than just "survive" on minimum daily requirements. I ask you, *minimum for whom*? Who wants to live a *minimum life*?

I suggest as a foundation (just in general and not for the purpose of treating disease) the following supplements: (The first three I consider especially important)

a. **Fish Oil** – containing EPA and DHA; the two omega–3 fatty acids necessary to reduce inflammation. It is estimated that we need to take enough fish oil every day in capsule or liquid form to receive 2000 mg of EPA, and 1000 mg of DHA, preferably obtained from small fish, like anchovies and sardines. (**Note:** EPA is a *physiologic* anti-inflammatory, and DHA is a *neurologic* anti-inflammatory.)

b. **Probiotics** – are essential to maintaining a normal level of bacteria in our intestines. Gut bacteria are responsible for digestion and B vitamin production, and they play a major role in our immune system. Antibiotics we've been prescribed and those we've ingested from our food and drinking water––think chlorine in drinking water––can deplete the normal bacterial levels in our gut. Therefore, refrigerated probiotics and fermented foods are essential to good health and normal bowel function.

c. **Vitamin D3** – is considered a hormone. Vitamin D is essential for proper immune function. 2000 IU to 10,000 IU is a daily minimum. Be sure to have your vitamin D levels tested when you have blood work done; it's essential to know what your levels are. (**Note:** 50 to 60 nanograms/milliliters is a good number to aim for.)

I consider the following three supplements a "must take" for every adult:

d. **Vitamin C** – 2000-3000 mg, every day. Vitamin C in general is essential to the health of our immune system, is an antioxidant, and is necessary to build and repair blood vessel tissues. If you have been diagnosed with a cancer syndrome, then I suggest IV Vitamin C supplementation of between 50,000 and 100,000 mg to be taken one to three times a week, as prescribed by your doctor.

e. **Multivitamin** – a high quality multivitamin, (4) capsules a day. Be sure the ingredients come from non-synthetic, naturally occurring substances—plant and animal, and are not from a factory or chemical lab—as much as possible.

f. **Calcium/Magnesium** – 2000 to 3000 mg of calcium taken from multiple sources—carbonate, citrate, gluconate, and phosphate, for example—and 1000 mg of magnesium, per day. Calcium and magnesium are often combined into one supplement. This combination is essential for good muscle tone and nerve function.

In addition to the supplements and nutrients above, it is important to use only glass cookware and storage products. Avoid plastic, Teflon, and aluminum as much as possible, as they contain toxins that could leach into your food.

When choosing what to eat, first ask yourself what would have been available to me 40,000 years ago, and let that serve as your template for how and what to eat from now on.

Be sure to drink adequate amounts of clean water every day; how much can vary from authority to authority, the external temperatures around you, and your level of activity. A minimum of six to eight glasses per day is often suggested, and it seems to be a good place to start.

Environmental

Our environments are made up of the air we breathe, the foods we eat, the sounds we hear, the odors and chemicals we come into contact with, and the people we surround ourselves with. Do you have Hard Rock or Beethoven playing on the radio? Ask yourself, are the sounds around me soothing? Are the noises from my TV and computer loud and annoying? What kind of video games are you playing? Are the people in my life healthy, positive, and honest? What do you surround yourself with? Is it healthy? Also make a "chemical check" of your work and home environment, looking for chemicals typically found in carpeting, processed woods, particleboards, and furniture, as these are insidious sources of toxins that silently affect many people.

Family/Community

We cannot change our family. In many cases, our family can be our rock. However, some people are toxic, negative, and abusive, and they can be in families, too. If these negative influences are in your life, even if they're family, let them go and do not associate with them further. Instead, create a support network of family and friends who will support you, be honest with you, and help you get stronger (as you do in turn for them). We are communal "animals" who find strength and support in groups. Find groups, communities, that support your core values. Do not try to face, handle, or overcome your syndrome alone. You must be "the decider," but you will do so much better when you have a community that cares about you and supports you.

> *We cannot live only for ourselves. A thousand fibers connect us with our fellow men; and among those fibers, as sympathetic threads, our actions run as causes, and they come back to us as effects.* – Herman Melville

Occupational

What are the hazards of your occupation? Do you overuse one side of your body? Do you sit all day? Are you exposed to chemicals or loud noises? Is your work something you love, or is it something you tolerate in order to put food on the table? Is your work in harmony with your core values? As we all know, life is short. If you're not doing work you enjoy and find value in, then do something else (or have something you enjoy that is supported by the occupation you need to tolerate). Robert Greenleaf in his essay, *Trustees as Servants,* asks the reader two questions, *whom do you serve* and *for what purpose?* Relative to occupations, these seem like good questions to ask. Remember, *happiness is a choice, not a result.* You can be satisfied with your occupation because of what it allows you to enjoy.

Look at the areas of your body or life that your occupation traumatizes, overworks, or abuses, and direct your exercise and stretching routines to compensate for the additional damage to that overworked area. Have a purpose for your workouts, know what areas need to be strengthened or stretched in response to trauma and what needs to be built up for the requirements of your work. If your work, in the final analysis, is too toxic to tolerate, change occupations or surroundings. No matter your age, your job could be killing you.

Spiritual

I am not speaking of being *religious* when I refer to *spiritual.* Spiritual can be looked upon as a faith in the inherent, inborn, something that gives us life and separates us from a dead body. It can be considered simply as a confidence in our *True Self.* Acknowledging, seeking, assisting that innate something with faith-based, introspective practices and disciplines, like meditation, prayer, and yoga, have been shown to a have a positive impact on our health (and they appear to be what we were designed to practice, anyway). Identify your core values, your *moral compass* and consider how you support and live by them. Explore your inner self with quiet introspection on a regular basis. Take time to reflect on how you are living, and what is important for your life.

Obviously, I have only touched on these topics and none of us will ever get all the areas in balance at one time. It is a lifetime process of slipping and checking, falling down and getting back up, and getting knocked off the tracks just to get back on them again. I suggest that you take this list of seven areas and write down everything that you could be doing to improve your life, in every area, and then pick one or two things to work on at a time. Next, review the list on a regular basis, adding new additions as you find them. Then, update the list, marking off what you feel you have completed. Keep this list with your Goals List, and picture yourself as the healthy, happy, person you want to be. (There is an *Action Steps* section at the end to help in this process.)

Know that adhering to a healthy program is especially difficult when attempting to go it alone. Almost all successful people have either a coach or committed listener; someone who will help them stay on the path to a goal or better life, and give them honest feedback. Consider hiring a coach to help you return to the healthier and better life you desire. A coach will listen and hear you differently than a friend or family member would. A coach will always ask the tough questions, asking you to look in the places you are afraid to look. Most of us will accept coaching more readily from a stranger than from a family member or friend because there are no past issues to cloud either persons perspective or judgment. In other words, a coach has no hidden agendas and isn't about just making you *"feel good."*

A coach will not allow you to live in excuses. A good coach *promises your promise.* This means they are giving you their word that you will attain *your goals,* even though they know they cannot directly affect the outcome. They will listen for the truth in your speaking and in your words, they will fight you for you, and they will have a *ruthless compassion* when it comes to helping you attain your goals. (*Ruthless compassion,* means that the coach understands that the action they are requesting is difficult and may be painful, but holds the person to their word, not accepting excuses, knowing that the good results will far exceed the temporary pain.)

Although at times, you might view your doctor as your coach, they are not the ideal person to have as a coach. Your doctor, while well intentioned, is invested in what *they think* is the right course of action to take, based on their professional perspective. However, you need a coach who will support what *you* think is the right course of action to take.

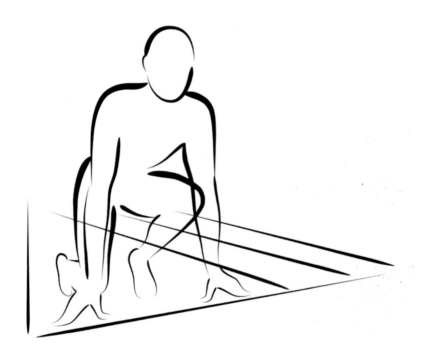

13 WHAT CAN I DO AND HOW DO I GET STARTED?

Nobody can go back and start a new beginning, but anyone can start today and make a new ending.

– Maria Robinson

As we get started, please note that I do not presume to have all the answers, not by any stretch of the imagination. No one has all the answers. I have some suggestions, based on what I have learned over my 45 years of caring for people in my practice who have presented with a myriad of dis-eases and conditions, and my personal life-experiences with melanoma and other life events. Each person is unique and different––historically, emotionally, and nutritionally.

The following are suggestions for where to begin (or that can help you continue on) your personal journey to discovering a better level of health. This is *your* journey. There is no one-size-fits-all solution for any health condition (despite the cookie-cutter, therapeutic approach of conventional medicine). In finding *your own solutions*, you can take (or leave) what I have to say, investigate additional resources, and/or consult with a functional medicine practitioner for adequate testing and additional guidance. *Apply what fits you, and leave the rest.*

In addition to the following list, you will notice an *Action List* at the end of this section and it is here that you can write down a few ideas to help you begin. In the following overview, I have placed asterisks (*/**) next to suggestions that I feel are most important. When working on your list, know that this is a process that no one gets *perfect,* or even completes. Begin with one or two topics then add more as you can.

14 MENTAL AND EMOTIONAL

1. **Be happy!** ***

2. Have someone with you at doctor's visits to ask the questions that you might forget to ask or won't ask. (Bring a family member, your coach, or a close friend you can trust who will be straight with you.) *

3. Hire a coach or have a committed listener (someone who will speak truth to you and assist you in staying on your path who will not promote their agenda). *

4. **Ask Questions and Question Everything** (including what you read in this book). *

5. Take charge and be responsible for your health and recovery. *

6. Admit your fears and move on. (Overcome and counter them with action steps. It is okay to be afraid, just don't allow fear to run your life. In other words, do not deny your fear but instead, understand it and move forward.) *

7. Make plans for the future (no matter the prognosis you are given). *

8. Live your life as *you* want to live it, and do that a day at a time.

9. Don't let your health/dis-ease become the focus of your existence. (When it comes to dealing with health issues, read books, search the Web, and ask others for help, BUT DO NOT let your health (dis-ease) become your focus. I've created a list of suggested links, books, and websites at the end of this booklet to help in your research.) *

10. Meditate, pray, and/or have your quiet time, every day.

11. Let go of the negative (including guilt, people, jobs, and bad situations).

12. Realize that you will go in and out of the Five Stages of Grief in response to your diagnosis ––Denial, Anger, Bargaining, Depression, and Acceptance. The rate at which you acknowledge and process through each will determine how quickly you return to your life.

13. Join a life-affirming support group focused on health and recovery (not disease and the latest pharmaceutical discovery).

14. Turn off the TV, computer, cell phone, and radio. (Allow your mind to rest.)

15. Keep a daily journal and/or write about your life. (Consider blogging or writing your life story.)

16. Repeat health-affirming affirmations as you go about your day, while at work, at play, and during exercise. (For example, you can repeat affirmations like, *I am vibrantly healthy, abundantly wealthy, and tremendously happy.*) You can make up your own, or use this one.

17. Read your Goals List every day.

15 PHYSICAL

1. Exercise aerobically 30 minutes a day, three to four hours a week. You can walk, dance, swim, or ride a bike, etc. *
2. Stretch or practice yoga, Pilates, or Tai Chi, every day.
3. Sleep a minimum of six to eight hours, every night.
4. Take naps when you need them.
5. Have spinal adjustments, as recommended.
6. Have acupuncture or meridian therapy, as suggested.
7. Have colonics or coffee enemas, as indicated.
8. Consider hyperbaric oxygen therapy treatments.

16 NUTRITIONAL

Programs may vary or even contradict these general recommendations; however, this is what I have found to be helpful for returning to good health:

1. Eliminate (or limit) grains, including all corn and corn products. *
2. Eliminate (or limit) dairy. *
3. Eliminate (or limit) refined sugar. *
4. Take IV therapies, including Vitamin C, Chelation, and Nutritional Support. As appropriate *
5. Drink juice made in a juicer (more concentrated, but less fiber) and/or smoothies (more fiber, but less concentrated) once a day or more. Use organic vegetables, especially greens and antioxidant fruits. *
6. Eat organic fruits and vegetables. Make organic fruits and vegetables more than 65 percent of your total, daily diet. *
7. Eat animal protein–– eggs, fish, and fowl plus range-fed and range-bled animal protein from herd animals––. Make animal protein less than 35 percent of your total, daily diet. *
8. Take supplements (as noted in the sections above and below).
9. Drink six to eight glasses of water a day.
10. Eat fermented foods frequently.
11. Do not eat fried foods.
12. Avoid trans–fats and genetically modified foods (GMOs).
13. Avoid legumes.

14. Eat *raw* nuts and other raw nut products——almonds, walnuts, almond milk, etc.
15. Use coconut oil and olive oil for cooking and as condiments.
16. Eat a fresh fruit or vegetable before every meal to introduce your body to a new way of eating.
17. Undertake a simple elimination diet, periodically.

17 FAMILY AND COMMUNITY

1. Do not isolate yourself. Have a community of friends and family for support. *

2. Do not allow people to be doom and gloom around you. *You are not dead.* *

3. Do not allow the conversations around you to center on your health or sickness. *

4. Allow family and friends to know what you are doing, and ask them for help if you need it.

5. Join a group for support and to grow and learn, and support your group, in return.

6. Reach out to and communicate with supportive friends and family.

7. Release negative people and situations from your life.

8. Love people in spite of how they behave, even if you dislike their behavior.

9. Associate with people who are open and honest, even if you do not like their truth.

10. Associate with people with similar values.

18 OCCUPATIONAL

1. See the purpose in your work/occupation, either in and of itself, or as a means to an end. *
2. If your work does not support your journey to health, change occupations.
3. Change your work environment so that it supports your life, goals and health.
4. Make your work *"play with a purpose."*
5. Exercise to counter any unhealthy physical affects from your work.
6. If you do not have an occupation, volunteer and serve others––people, animals, plants, church, community, and/or family. Be engaged and involved in actions that are satisfying to you. (Be selfless, but not at the expense of your health.)
7. *Ask yourself, whom do I serve and for* what purpose?

19 SPIRITUAL

1. What is your life's purpose? (Write it out.) *

2. What is a perfect life to you? (Write it out, in detail.) *

3. What are your core life-guiding values? (Write them down.) *

4. Be grateful for everything. Develop an attitude of gratitude. *

5. Acknowledge and reach out to your Higher Power, whomever/whatever you envision that to be.

6. Worship, pray, or meditate. (Do whatever nurtures you and your Spirit, daily.)

7. Simply put, have faith in something.

8. Listen to your inner voice (not your ego, fearful and self-important self, but your inner true self).

9. Savor where you are now, every moment of the day.

10. Appreciate the people in your life.

11. Take time to read something uplifting, every day.

20 ENVIRONMENTAL

1. Surround yourself with positive, inspiring people. *
2. Drink clean water. (Have a filter or buy filtered water.)
3. Breathe clean air. (Install filters and/or humidifiers to allow clean air to flow.)
4. Surround yourself with images and colors that you find positive and inspiring.
5. Turn off the TV.
6. Listen to uplifting music.
7. Surround yourself in situations where you can grow mentally and spiritually.
8. Avoid eating genetically modified foods and plants (GMOs).
9. Use glass cookware and storage containers.
10. Avoid personal hygiene products that contain chemicals.
11. Avoid aerosol products.
12. Check your home for chemicals, mold, and other toxins.

21 IN SUMMARY

Time is the consumer and we are the food

Everyone I know who has returned to a vibrant state of health has changed their diet. And almost everyone I know who has been diagnosed with a cancer syndrome that regained their health, included juicing or making smoothies (and consumed them daily). In addition, those with any type of syndrome began to exercise or continued to exercise, faithfully. (I say *faithfully*, because I think exercising *religiously* must mean that the person talks about it a lot, and might do some on Sundays.) And, without a doubt, every person I know who has recovered or improved significantly had a positive, affirming attitude about their life. (Not a rah-rah, superficial show, but a quiet, inner sense of, *everything happens exactly as it is supposed to, and that's okay.*)

Those who regained their vibrant health had a certainty of purpose, an inner calm; they were not lost in fear and despair. This is not to say that they did not have moments of uncertainty, fear, anger, anxiety, or depression, but these emotions were *temporary down times* for them inside the context of their bigger picture of life. Many also had a coach. The person may not have had the title "coach", but there was someone helping them who acted like a coach. That person was committed to helping them return to more vibrant health.

Please know that we are all on a similar journey, and fundamentally, we all have similar choices to make in regard to our health. I don't have all the answers. I just have suggestions that I have found to be true for me (personally), and for many that I've cared for. All of these suggestions may not be right for you; however, if you are facing a health crisis, you need to make some lifestyle changes, and the transition will be smoother if you have support from a coach, your family, and/or your community. Hopefully, this book will help direct you to finding *YOUR* answers for health and bring balance to your life.

Insanity has been defined as, *doing the same thing over and over again, expecting a different result*. Bottom line? Don't act insane.

22 CLOSING SUGGESTIONS

Before you begin taking action steps, it is important to remember that change is an ongoing process. The process of change can be described as an endless spiral, like a Slinky toy. According to Peter Senge, author of *The Fifth Discipline; The Art and Practice of Learning Organization*, the process of change is a continuous cycle of Dialogue to Insight to Action to Reflection that returns back to Dialogue. Many become stuck in the Dialogue to Insight loop (all talk and lots of dreaming), or in a continuously same Action loop (in a rut; *a grave with both ends tapered*), or trapped in an ongoing Reflection loop (herein lies *guilt*).

Positive change requires conscious and continuous advancement through the cycle of change in order to be effective. With this in mind, take a few moments to reconsider the questions you were asked in the beginning, then begin planning your next action steps in your return to health. Do not look back at your previous answers until you have answered these questions again to see if anything has shifted for you.

Again, pay attention to your first thoughts as you ask yourself these questions, and understand there are no right or wrong answers:

1. What does the diagnosis your health provider gave you mean to you?
2. What does your diagnosis stop you from doing (in all areas of your life)?
3. What do you want to be able to do? (Dream big! Think in short-term, long-term, family, vocation, and avocation, etc.)

4. What are you doing now that is not in balance with your values?

5. What is most important to you?

6. What are you afraid of?

7. What are you willing to do?

If you are going to succeed in restoring your health, it is vitally important that your actions align with *what you want* in your life, not what someone else thinks your life should be. I believe if you honestly answer these questions, you can better prioritize your next steps and be more willing to commit to the necessary actions needed to make the rest of your life more fulfilling, happier, and more satisfying for you. Remember, **YOU *are in charge!***

You are loved and cherished, dearly, forever.
You have nothing to fear.
There is nothing you can do wrong.

– Proof of Heaven, by E. Alexander, M.D.

23 YOU ARE IN CHARGE

Whatever you can do, or dream you can, begin it. Boldness has genius,
magic, and power in it. Begin it now.

– Goethe

Where to begin? You now have all of these suggestions, ideas, and "cures" for what to do. You might want to try them all, or you might not want to do anything but exchange your life with someone else, ask for a do-over, or just sit there feeling sorry for yourself. Where to start? What to do first? Is the problem your attitude, diet, environment, or job? As my youngest child used to cry, "I don't know what to do." A good overall place to begin and simplify your efforts is to consolidate what you need to do, down to the simplest terms––*eat well, move well, and think well.* Inside of this simple concept, the following sections are provided to give you an opportunity to list action steps to help you get moving in a healthier direction.

Starting is more than 50 percent of the battle, and this workbook is intended to help you get started. It is important to understand that we will never get it 100 percent right, and that we will never truly know if we are doing the right thing, 100 percent. We can only do the best we can do in this moment in time, and continue to live our lives to the fullest, as best we can.

The following action steps are divided into seven sections that correspond with the seven areas of major influence in our lives, as mentioned earlier. I suggest picking no more than three action steps at a time. Focus on making your action steps a part of your life for thirty days, or if possible, completing a step before taking on the next step. Some actions can be lumped into one, like adding supplements to your diet and then specifying which supplements that would be. And some actions you will start that were never intended to end because they have indefinite points of completion. Other actions might be only for a few weeks, months, or even a year or two. Also remember that you will probably fall off the horse more than once. You might feel as if you've failed to accomplish your goal or action step, *so why even try*? Get back up and start again or continue on. None of us gets it perfect the first time; it usually it takes practice, repetition, and time.

A technique that can help you choose action steps and follow through with the steps you've chosen is setting SMART Goals. S.M.A.R.T is an acronym for Specific, Measurable (or Meaningful), Achievable (or Attainable), Relevant (or Reasonable), and Time specific (or by when). When choosing your action steps or goals, use the S.M.A.R.T. system to be clear about what you want to accomplish. For example, ask yourself, "S" – What specifically are you going to do or accomplish? "M" – What are the mileposts that will show you that you are moving toward your desired finish, and are these mileposts clearly measurable? "A" – Be certain that you can accomplish the goal, and that it is not some pie-in-the-sky wishful thinking as you might have done in the past. You may need to create interim goals to achieve a bigger, less immediately achievable or seemingly impossible goal. "R" – Does the goal relate to your overall desired outcome, and is it within the realm of possibility? (For example, winning the lottery is possible, but certainly not a good retirement plan.) "T" – Give yourself a "by when" asking yourself, within what timeframe is this to be accomplished by? (For example, I will start walking consistently three times a week for 30 minutes a day on Wednesdays, or on ___/___/___").

Please be aware that each area may have a subset in other areas. For example, in the area called *Physical* you will see the subset, *Exercise*, which is meant to apply to your whole body and includes aerobic exercise, general muscle tone, and general stretching. *Exercise* also applies to the area, *Occupational*; however in this area, subset *Exercise* is used to help you identify the areas you need to build, loosen, or address in response to the tasks you must perform and the trauma caused by your occupation. Sitting at a computer all day, using one arm repetitively (for example, as a carpenter does), standing on your feet for hours at a time, and lifting or twisting repeatedly are all examples of how one area may be overworked or stressed that would require specific stretches and exercises to reduce and minimize the damage from your occupation.

Finally, before we continue, I recommend that you take a few moments and decide what it is that you are *NOT* willing to do, give up, or change, and write them below. Let's get these out of the way so you aren't trying to do something that you will probably fail at because you really do not want to change or do it. For me, I will not have chemotherapy or radiation, and I will not give up my daily coffee. I enjoy a couple of cups of coffee every day. That is that. I choose also not to expose my body to unnecessary radiation or minimally effective toxic chemicals and drugs. These are things I will not do and will not change. You don't have to have a reason; it's just what's right for you, right now. Know that someday in the far-off future, it is possible that you might change your mind, but for now these three things are not something that you are willing to give up or to do, period. As a coach, knowing the things that you are positive you will never change helps me avoid nagging you about something you are not willing to do, so this saves us both time and energy.

Let's Get Started!

List three things that you will not likely ever change, give up, or do:

1.

_____

2.

_____

3.

_____

Now that these unchangeable items have been identified, let's head into the other direction by asking, *what ARE you willing to do?* The following sections are not in any particular order. Feel free to pick and choose your three action steps from any of the seven areas.

My Spiritual Action Steps

What do I need to do to improve my connection with a "Higher Power", and what do I need to stop doing? How do I find inner calm? What are my values?

Applying spiritual action steps is a process that's usually more personal to most people. For you, it could mean finding some quiet time, listening to your inner self, taking time for prayer (or making life a prayer), and identifying your life-guiding values.

List below everything that you could do, or need to stop doing, in order to improve your environment. Place the starting date in front of the choice(s) you make. Remember to choose *no more than three* at a time:

____/___/___ _____

____/___/___ _____

____/___/___ _____

____/___/___ _____

____/___/___ _____

____/___/___ _____

My Nutritional Action Steps

What do I need to do to improve my diet, and what do I need to stop doing?

Here are some ideas to help you get started on the right track: drink fruit and vegetable juice/smoothies; limit your diet to less than 20 percent refined grains; limit or eliminate dairy; choose organic foods; drink six to eight glasses of water a day; take fish oil (2000 mg EPA/1000 mg DHA) daily; make 65 percent of your diet fruits and vegetables and 35 percent range-fed proteins; take supplements; eliminate plastics, aluminum, and Teflon from cooking and food storage; cut out refined sugars; have a raw fresh fruit or vegetable before each meal.

List below everything that you could do, or need to stop doing, to improve your nutritional condition. Place the starting date in front of the choice(s) you make. Remember to choose *no more than three* at a time:

____/___/___ _____

____/___/___ _____

____/___/___ _____

____/___/___ _____

____/___/___ _____

____/___/___ _____

My Family/Community Action Steps

What do I need to do to improve my relationships with my community/family and what do I need to stop doing?

Family is impossible to change; however, *you can* ignore or remove yourself from toxic family members. Ask yourself, are the people who you surround yourself with supportive of who you want to become? Do you gain support from the people in your life, and do you support them, as well? Who is in your community? Do your have a coach or a committed listener? Do you have a support group or community?

List below everything that you could do, or need to stop doing, to improve your family and community environments. Place the starting date in front of the choice(s) you make. Remember to choose *no more than three* at a time:

_____/___/___ _____

_____/___/___ _____

_____/___/___ _____

_____/___/___ _____

_____/___/___ _____

_____/___/___ _____

My Occupational/Avocational Action Steps

What do I need to do to improve my vocational life, and what do I need to stop doing?

Here are some questions you can ask yourself to help find some answers, like, is your job your *dream job*? Is your occupation something you enjoy, like *play with a purpose*? What areas of your body do you need to rebuild and/or protect because of your occupation? What is your workplace environment like (physically, chemically, and emotionally)? Does your occupation support your higher purpose in life, and does it represent your core values?

List below everything that you could do or need to stop doing in order to improve your occupational/avocational environment. Place the starting date in front of the choice(s) you make. Remember to choose *no more than three* at a time:

___/___/___ _____

___/___/___ _____

___/___/___ _____

___/___/___ _____

___/___/___ _____

___/___/___ _____

My Mental/Emotional Action Steps

What do I need to do to improve my attitude and my creative stress?
What do I need to stop doing?

Here are some suggestions to help you discover action steps you can take in this area, like setting short, intermediate, and long-term goals, and review them daily; meditate; turn off your electronics; make a bucket list; make plans for the future; avoid certain people (_____); forgive yourself and others; have your quiet time every day; release any guilt you might be having over past situations (_____); visualize your goals daily; identify your life purpose; write out a description of your perfect life; write or journal on a daily or weekly basis.

List below everything that you could do or need to stop doing in order to improve your mental and emotional state. Place the starting date in front of the choice(s) you make. Remember to choose *no more than three* at a time:

_____/___/___ _____

_____/___/___ _____

_____/___/___ _____

_____/___/___ _____

_____/___/___ _____

My Environmental Action Steps

What do I need to do to improve my environment, and what do I need to stop doing?

Your environment includes things like, the air you breathe; the foods you eat; the liquids you drink; the people you surround yourself with; how you entertain yourself; the noise that surrounds you; the chemicals you are exposed to; your support community; and your opportunities to rest.

List below everything that you could do or need to stop doing to improve your environment. Place the starting date in front of the choice(s) you make. Remember to choose *no more than three* at a time:

_____/___/___ _____

_____/___/___ _____

_____/___/___ _____

_____/___/___ _____

_____/___/___ _____

_____/___/___ _____

My Physical Action Steps

What do I need to do to improve my physical condition, and what do I need to stop doing?

Here are some suggestions to help you improve your physical condition, like do 30 minutes of aerobic activity, every day; get seven to eight hours of sleep, every night; stretch every major area of your body daily (Tai Chi, yoga, and meditation can help); have regular spinal adjustments; improve your posture; do not remain in one position for longer than an hour at a time; 15 minutes of whole body vibration a day.

List below everything that you could do or need to stop doing to improve your physical condition. Place the starting date in front of the choice(s) you make. Remember to choose *no more than three* at a time:

_____/___/___ _____

_____/___/___ _____

_____/___/___ _____

_____/___/___ _____

_____/___/___ _____

_____/___/___ _____

APPENDIX

Following is a list of the supplements, therapies, and nutrients that I have used to improve my own health. Some I recommend for general health support, and others I believe are important for anyone with an immune condition or who has been diagnosed with a cancer syndrome. Of course, these are in addition to following a diet that is 65 percent fresh organic fruits and vegetables, and 35 percent range-fed and range-bled proteins, drinking adequate amounts of clean water, avoiding dairy, and reducing your intake of grains on a daily basis. In addition I have listed some resources that I have found helpful in my journey to better health

You should be advised that this is not a "cookbook cure" for any one condition; instead, these are suggestions to help you begin to change your health, and topics to help you understand your options for treatment when discussing your dis-ease or condition with your health care provider. (Remember; throwing a bunch of vitamins, herbs, and supplements at a condition without the benefit of educated guidance, investigation, and coaching, is never a good plan of action.)

Supplements and Nutrients – Below is a list of what I take:

(Supplements should be taken to support the whole day and not taken all at once. I take mine twice per day. The dosages below are the total amount in a day and are divided into two times per day except where indicated.)

A. **Supplements** (A basic list, suggested for general health):
1. Refrigerated Probiotics 100 billion CFU– (1) dose in the a.m., and (1) dose in the p.m. *
2. Fish Oil – sufficient to supply 2,000 mg of EPA and 1,000 mg of DHA* *
3. Vitamin D3 – 2000 IU to 4000 IU. (I was taking 20,000 IU * daily, until I raised my blood levels up to between 50 ng/ml and 60 ng/ml.)
4. CoQ10 – 200 to 400 mg *
5. Vitamin E – to be taken in the delta-tocotrienol 500 mg form, not in the tocopherol form, a day *
6. Multivitamin – a *quality* multivitamin, four to six capsules.
7. Vitamin C – 2000 to 4000 mg.
8. Green Tea or Green Tea Extract 1000 mg.
9. Raw Local Honey – (1) tablespoon.

B. **Inflammatory and Autoimmune Conditions** (in addition to the basic list above):
1. Breakfast Smoothie – including kale, broccoli, carrots, ginger, blueberries, pineapple, black seed oil, raw honey, organic apple cider vinegar, and coconut water, making a 32 oz. serving, every day. Sometimes I'll toss in an apple, asparagus, beet, banana, or other fruits and vegetables for variety. (This is *absolutely essential* in helping you regain your optimal health!) (**Note:** There are many other vegetables and fruits that you can use in addition to what I've listed here.) **
2. Modified Citrus Pectin – 6.4 gm. a day for healthy cell growth and to rebuild your immune system. *
3. Vitamin D3 – 20,000 IU *.

4. Turmeric – (2) capsules, three times a day (for an approximate total of 900 mg a day). *

5. Black Seed Oil – (1) tablespoon a day (in smoothie).

6. Quercetin – 1000 mg.

C. **Cancer Syndromes** (in addition to List B, above):

1. Vitamin C in IV Form – 50,0000 to 100,000 mg, one to two times a week (three times in the beginning). *

2. Mistletoe Injections – purchased through Canadian, Mexican, and European clinics and/or doctors. Used to help prevent metastasis. Mistletoe injections are labeled as Helixor or Iscador (Weleda)* Take as directed by prescribing physician.

3. Hemp Oil – legal in many states, including Washington State. It can be used internally, and/or applied to external lesions* (For more information, do Web searches for "Phoenix Tears.") *

4. Naltrexone 4.5 mg – an off-label drug for tumor reduction and a general anti-inflammatory.

5. Graviola (Soursop) Tea – use daily as a fruit, in smoothies, juice, or as a tea. *

6. Mushroom Extract – made from shiitake or rishi mushrooms. Use will be based on what is appropriate for your dis-ease.

D. **Melanoma** (in addition to supplements/nutrients in List C):

1. Chaga Mushroom – in lieu of shitake or rishi mushrooms. 1600 mg.

2. Melatonin 20 mg – suggested use is specific to melanoma. One at night.

E. **Miscellaneous:**

1. Hyperbaric Oxygen – three to ten therapy sessions after every surgery. *

2. Chiropractic Adjustments – one to four adjustments, per month.

A. **Treatments to Consider:**

1. IV Chelation Therapy – especially recommended where there has been heavy metal toxicity exposure and in treating immune dis-eases. *

2. Thyroid Testing – in addition to standard blood work testing. Regulating your thyroid is essential with autoimmune disorders.

3. "Gut test" for good bacteria

4. Vitamin B-17/Laetrile – as directed by prescribing physician.

5. Sleep Apnea – if you have trouble sleeping

6. Coffee Enemas and/or Colon Hydrotherapy – as directed by physician and condition.

Suggested Reading

1. *Knockout*, by Suzanne Somers. Three Rivers Press, New York, NY. (2009)

2. *Naturopathic Oncology; An Encyclopedia Guide for Patients and Doctors*, by Dr. Neil McKinney, B.Sc., N.D. Liaison Press, Vancouver BC, Canada. (2010)

3. *Anti-Cancer; A New Way of Life*, by David Servan-Schreiber, M.D., Ph.D. Penguin Group, New York, NY. (2009)

4. *The Disease Delusion; Conquering the Causes of Chronic Illness for a Healthier, Longer, and Happier Life*, by Dr. Jeffrey S. Bland and Dr. Mark Hyman. Harper-Collins, New York, NY. (2014)

5. *Cancer; Step Outside the Box*, by Ty M. Bollinger. Infinity 510^2 Partners, Miami, FL. (2006)

6. *Outsmart Your Cancer; Alternative Non-Toxic Treatments That Work*, by Tanya Harter Pierce. ThoughtWorks Publishing, Lake Tahoe, CA. (2009)

7. *The Wellness Prevention Paradigm*, by James L. Chestnut, B.Ed., M.Sc., D.C. The Wellness Practice Global Self Health Corp., Victoria, BC (2010)

8. *Grain Brain: The Surprising Truth about Wheat, Carbs, and Sugar; Your Brain's Silent Killers,* by David Perlmutter and Kristin Loberg. Little, Brown and Company, New York, NY. (2013)

9. *Healing the Gerson Way; Defeating Cancer and Other Chronic Diseases*, by Charlotte Gerson, Beata Bishop, Joanne Shwed and Abram Hoffer. Totality Books, Carmel, CA. (2009)

10. *Defeat Cancer; 15 Doctors of Integrative & Naturopathic Medicine Tell You How*, by Connie Strasheim. BioMed Publishing Group, So. Lake Tahoe, CA (2011)

11. *Cancer Report: The Latest Research – How Thousands are Achieving Permanent Recoveries* (2005), by W. Douglas Brodie and John R. Voell. Change Your World Press, Reno, NV (004)

Suggested Diets to Consider

1. *The Paleo Diet; Lose Weight and Get Healthy by Eating the Food You Were Designed to Eat, Revised Edition,* Loren Cordain, Ph.D.

2. *Gerson Therapy Handbook,* Gerson Institute

3. *Fasting and Eating for Health,* Joel Fuhrman, M.D.

4. *Healing the Gerson Way: Defeating Cancer and Other Chronic Diseases,* Charlotte Gerson, Beata Bishop, Joanne Shwed, and Abram Hoffer

5. *Hoxsey Therapy: When Natural Cures for Cancer Became Illegal; the Autobiography of Harry Hoxsey,* N.D., Harry Hoxsey, N.D.

Resources for Inspiration

1. *Love, Medicine and Miracles,* by Bernie Siegel, M.D.

2. *Enjoy Every Sandwich; Living Each Day as If it Were Your Last,* by Lee Lipsenthal, M.D.

3. *Proof of Heaven; A Neurosurgeon's Journey into the Afterlife,* by Eben Alexander, M.D.

4. *E-Squared; Nine Do-It-Yourself Energy Experiments,* by Pam Grout

5. *The War of Art; Break Through the Blocks and Win Your Inner Creative Battles,* by Steven Pressfield and Shawn Coyne

Online Resources

A. Products

1. Mistletoe; Helixor http://www.helixor.com/integrative-cancer-therapy/

2. Mushroom Products http://www.jhsnp.com/products/chaga-mushroom/

3. Phoenix Tears; Hemp Oil http://phoenixtears.ca/dosage-information/

4. Modified Citrus Pectin http://www.econugenics.com/shop-by-product/pectasol-c-modified-citrus-pectin-main/

5. Plants that Cure http://www.thehealersbible.com/fruits---vegetables---plants--trees-that-cure.html

6. Turmeric Resources http://www.tattvasherbs.com/index

7. Vitamin E and Tocotrienols http://www.acgrace.com/unique-e-vitamin-e/unique-e-tocotrienols/

8. Avemar http://www.avemar.com/what_is_avemar

B. Suggested Reading

1. Honey http://www.slideshare.net/jflariviere/honey-a-promising-anticancer-agent

2. Graviola/Soursop http://www.greenmedinfo.com/blog/fruit-extract-10000-times-better-chemo

3. Mistletoe Studies http://www.cancer.gov/cancertopics/pdq/cam/mistletoe/HealthProfessional/page5

4. Hemp Oil and Other Suggestions http://organic-health.us/cancer/cannabis-hemp-oil.shtml

5. CBD in Hemp Oil http://www.projectcbd.org/

6. Gerson Diet http://gerson.org/gerpress/the-gerson-therapy/

7. Natural Lifestyles Network http://naturallifestyle.net/profiles/The-Center-for-Advancement-in-Cancer-Education-135

8. Ketogenic Diet http://www.cbn.com/cbnnews/healthscience/2012/december/starving-cancer-ketogenic-diet-a-key-to-recovery/

9. Cancer Control Society http://www.cancercontrolsociety.com/

10. Radiation and Increased Cancer http://www.greenmedinfo.com/blog/study-radiation-therapy-can-make-cancers-30x-more-malignant

11. Low-dose Naltrexone http://www.lowdosenaltrexone.org/; http://www.ldnresearchtrust.org/

12. Will Smith on Success (Inspirational) https://www.youtube.com/watch?v=q5nVqeVhgQE

C. Integrative and Alternative Medical Clinics – There are more good clinics that work with people with dis-ease syndromes. Here are a few to point you in the right direction:

1. Dr. Neil McKinney http://vitalvictoria.ca/
2. Mt. Rainier Clinic http://mtrainierclinic.com/index.html
3. Dr. Burzynski http://burzynskipatientgroup.org/jessica-kerfoot
4. Dr. Nicholas Gonzales http://www.dr-gonzalez.com/index.htm
5. Israeli Cancer Center http://israel21c.org/health/israeli-lab-therapy-treats-melanoma-with-the-plasma-of-autoimmune-disease-patients/
6. Hoxsey Clinic http://www.hoxseybiomedical.com/
7. Dr. Contreras http://www.oasisofhope.com/
8. Dr. Rodrigo Rodriguez http://www.biocarehospital.com/

REFERENCES

1. Pg. 6 – YERVOY® (generic ipilimumab), the latest medical treatment for melanoma, has a 7–10 percent response rate. http://www.ncbi.nlm.nih.gov/pmc/articles/PMC3799873/; http://www.ncbi.nlm.nih.gov/pmc/articles/PMC3700777/

2. Pg. 9 – Statistically, approximately 70% of the people diagnosed with Stage IV melanoma do not live five years from the time of diagnosis. – American Joint Committee on Cancer. 2002 P. 209-220

3. Pg. 13 – Some literature estimates that trying to destroy cancer cells with chemotherapy or radiation causes up to a 350% or more increase in cancer cell activity. - Dean Black, Ph.D., *Health At the Crossroads*. Tapestry Press, 1988. (P. 49)

4. Pg. 13 – *Many who have been diagnosed with most other forms of cancer and follow the traditional chemotherapy and radiation protocols do not live past 10 years.* http://www.naturalnews.com/030347_chemotherapy_risks.html http://www.reuters.com/article/2010/07/13/us-cancer-childhood-idUSTRE66C65120100713

5. Pg. 16 – Democritus countered that Hippocrates was espousing a religion and that only through scientific understanding of our body's physical makeup could health be maintained. Later, Benjamin Rush, M.D., a signer of the Declaration of Independence, expanded Democritus' position with the comment that it was the art

of the physician to take the role of healing out of nature's hands. *
– Dean Black, Ph.D., *Health At the Crossroads*. Tapestry Press,
1988 (P. 14, 30, & 33)

6. Pg. 19 – ...it however is not effective in changing the mortality rate
   or the incidence rate of the flu. *
   http://onlinelibrary.wiley.com/doi/10.1002/14651858.CD001269.p
   ub4/full

   http://www.ncbi.nlm.nih.gov/pubmed?orig_db=PubMed&cmd=Se
   arch&term=%22Archives+of+pediatrics+%26+adolescent+medicin
   e%22[Jour]+AND+2008%2F10[pdat]+AND+Szilagyi[author]

   http://www.ncbi.nlm.nih.gov/pubmed?orig_db=PubMed&cmd=Se
   arch&term=%22The+Lancet+infectious+diseases%22[Jour]+AND
   +658[page]+AND+2007[pdat

   http://www.ncbi.nlm.nih.gov/pubmed?orig_db=PubMed&cmd=Se
   arch&term=American+journal+of+respiratory+and+critical+care+
   medicine[Jour]+AND+527[page]+AND+2008[pdat

7. Pg. 21 – Statin medications are stated to be effective in reducing the
   incidence of heart events by 50%.
   http://www.theheart.org/article/1093495.do
   http://www.ncbi.nlm.nih.gov/pmc/articles/PMC2644034/
   http://www.ncbi.nlm.nih.gov/pmc/articles/PMC3023269/

8. http://www.westonaprice.org/modern-diseases/dangers-of-statin-
   drugs-what-you-havent-been-told-about-popular-cholesterol-
   lowering-medicines/

9. Pg. 22 – Publication Bias
   http://www.medpagetoday.com/MeetingCoverage/PRC/15964
   http://www.medscape.com/viewarticle/829866?src=wnl_edit_spe
   col#vp_2
   http://journals.plos.org/plosmedicine/article?id=10.1371/journal.p
   med.0020124

10. Pg. 22 – It has been estimated that up to 50% of currently
    published material has some degree of publication bias ranging

from minor human error to out-and-out fraud.
http://www.medpagetoday.com/MeetingCoverage/PRC/15964
http://www.medscape.com/viewarticle/829866?src=wnl_edit_spe
col#vp_2
http://journals.plos.org/plosmedicine/article?id=10.1371/journal.p
med.0020124

11. Pg. 27 - They become genetically adapted to the chemical toxins from the chemotherapy (gene amplification) - Dean Black, Ph.D., *Health At the Crossroads.* Tapestry Press, 1988. (P. 10 & 49)

12. Pg. 28 – It is also important to note that a study in *Clinical Oncology* in 2004 found that with only a few exceptions, chemotherapy caused only a 2.1% impact on 5-year survival rates. - *The Contribution of Cytotoxic Chemotherapy to 5 Years Survival in Adult Malignancies* – Graeme Morgan, Robyn Ward, Michael Barton. *Clinical Oncology (2004) 16: 549-560 doi: 10.1016/j.clon.2004.06.007*

13. Pg. 28 – And it should also be noted that in a survey of 118 doctors from McGill University who were involved in cancer treatment and research, 75 percent indicated they would not have chemotherapy if diagnosed with some form of cancer.
*http://www.naturalnews.com/036054_chemotherapy_physicians_toxicit
y.html*

ABOUT THE AUTHOR

Dr. Bomonti graduated from The National College of Chiropractic (now National University of Health Sciences) in 1968 and finished his internship in 1969. He was in practice with his mentor, Dr. Lee Arnold, for the next five years and in 1976 he moved to his wife's home State of Washington. He has been in private practice in Puyallup, Washington since 1976 and has been actively involved in his community and his profession. He has served as president of various civic organizations including the Puyallup Chamber of Commerce and has served for 13 years on the Advisory Board of the local YMCA. He was also active in the Washington Chiropractic Association, Puget Sound Chiropractic Resource and the Washington State Chiropractic Association, receiving multiple awards for his service. He has participated in numerous professional and personal educational programs over the years, endeavoring to improve his care to his patients. In 2002 he created a ten week personal and health transformation program called "Access to Change" which made it possible to help many people regain control over their lives and their health. Additionally, he has coached literally hundreds of people over the past forty plus years in their attempts to enhance their lives and improve their health.

Enjoying life within the beauty of the Great Northwest, Dr. Bomonti is married to his wife of 46 years, Jan, and they have two grown daughters. He enjoys playing golf in his spare time as well as reading on a variety of subjects.

Dr. Bomonti is available through the Mt. Rainier Clinic in Gig Harbor, Washington (mtrainierclinic.com or youareincharge.net) for health care services, life/health coaching and speaking opportunities.

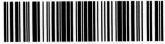

Made in the USA
Columbia, SC
19 April 2019